HEALTH CARE: CAN THERE BE EQUITY?

HEALTH CARE: Can There Be Equity?
The United States, Sweden, and England

ODIN W. ANDERSON, Ph.D.

Center for Health Administration Studies
University of Chicago

A Wiley-Interscience Publication

JOHN WILEY & SONS, New York · London · Sydney · Toronto

Library of Congress Cataloging in Publication Data

Anderson, Odin Waldemar, 1914–
  Health care.

  Bibliography: p.
  1. Medical care—United States.   2. Medical care—
Sweden.   3. Medical care—Great Britain.   I. Title.
[DNLM: 1. Community health services.   WA 525 A548h
1972]

RA395.A3A6   362.1   72-7449
ISBN 0-471-02760-X

Printed in the United States of America

10 9 8 7 6 5 4 3 2 1

Foreword

The continued search for better methods of caring for the sick and lack of consensus about the best organization make this book timely and important. Evaluation of how and why health services in the United States and two other countries have developed are here explored with enlightenment and an objectivity seldom vouchsafed and badly needed in this emotional, one might say, bloody, field. The good judgments expressed flow from a lifetime of well chosen research as a medical sociologist and health services generalist.

Organization of medical care in the United States has been described as chaotic, a nonsystem. There are those who promise that problems of cost and quality will be solved if some new method, organization, or system is adopted. The search for quick solution goes on and could lead to ill advised national decisions.

Since good health, as the author points out, is so ill defined and undefinable, the comparison of structure, staffing, and use of health services in three countries with similar cultures is useful, particularly so since two of the countries have universal health insurance. The comparison should give directions for improving care in each country, but especially in the United States at this juncture.

The organization of medical care has moved to greater structure and control through national health insurance in England and Sweden. More control is recommended to accompany national health insurance here.

v

Such insurance has the great merit of providing a floor of medical care to all with little or no payment at time of service, but authority accompanies it. Under the British system controls permitted some containment of expenditure, though this is less true in Sweden. The extent of regulation in proposals for a nationalized system is a major issue here.

The drive for more control and different organization proposed for the United States, to some degree, can be evaluated after the fact in these two countries. Governmental systems in England and Sweden have many of the problems most criticized in the United States with its "nonsystem." The values of a governmental system are both understated and overstated. Such a system with detailed regulation would not necessarily contain costs nor solve other problems—indeed, it would exacerbate some.

This valuable study suggests what different universal health insurance systems will and will not accomplish. This is important for the United States as the Congress debates policy. Too great regulation or compromises required to secure passage could bring limited values and great problems that study of experience elsewhere might avoid.

This book represents more than 10 years of search for understanding of health services in England and Sweden. Data have been collected and examined for comparability between the three countries. Results are presented, qualified, and cautiously interpreted. It is timely and should significantly affect public policy that will shape that vital human service—namely, care of the sick. Finally, the value of international comparisons of health services so well demonstrated in this book should encourage continuing joint study in the three countries.

GEORGE BUGBEE

Genesee Depot, Wisconsin
April 1971

Preface

This book has been a long time in the making. For some time my staff and I have been gathering an extensive set of sources and information on health care in the United States, Sweden, and Great Britain. Our starting point was the official reports on facilities, personnel, programs, and costs over time in all three countries. In addition, I made myself thoroughly familiar with each country's formal studies of the health services from population consumption patterns to reports on organization and delivery methods. Many will be cited in due course.

Another important source of information is the research I have been associated with directly. In planning the third of a series of surveys of a sample of households nationwide for 1963,[1] I proposed to appropriate authorities in Sweden and Great Britain that they collaborate with the Center for Health Administration Studies and the National Opinion Research Center, both at the University of Chicago, in concurrent studies on use and expenditure patterns. This collaboration would have provided comparative data using very much the same methods for three countries with varying organizational and financing mechanisms for their health services.

At the time this proposal was made, 1960, the British Ministry of

---

[1] Andersen and Anderson (1967). Previous surveys resulted in Anderson and Feldman (1956) and Anderson, Collette, and Feldman (1963). A fourth study covering calendar year 1970 is now under way.

Health was more interested in some type of operations research regarding hospital efficiency than in a survey of how the population used services. The Swedish authorities in the National Medical Board were interested in this type of population survey, however. That country appeared ready to take a comprehensive look at its health services, and a social survey was regarded as a useful approach.[2]

A fruitful collaboration between research staffs of the Department of Social Medicine, University of Uppsala, and the staffs of the Center for Health Administration Studies and the National Opinion Research Center resulted in comparative surveys in the two countries. Data from these surveys are drawn on in the course of this book.[3] Fortunately, some data of this nature are now available for England and Wales. Although they are not strictly comparable to the Swedish and American data, it is possible to make some gross comparisons in patterns of use.

Another source of information is a rather extensive reading of the social, political, economic, and historical literature of the three countries. It is a truism that the health services of a country develop in relation to a certain sociopolitical-economic matrix. The sheer technology of a modern health service creates certain organizational patterns and personnel types regardless of the overall social system, but some of the organizational and personnel differences, and particularly the problem-solving styles of different countries, affect the developmental patterns. Hence I felt the need to review this type of literature.

Finally, I interviewed 40 to 50 "leaders" each in Sweden and Great Britain in politics, academia, health service administration, business management, labor organization, the various health professions, and in key positions in the official health bureaucracies. My questioning was directed mainly to the "problems and issues" in the health services as they saw them. These interviews were hardly systematic in an interview schedule concept; rather, they were open ended for the purpose of getting a feel for the general atmosphere. Also, I was thoroughly familiar with the health services in each country. It was not necessary to carry out interviews in the United States in the same sense, because of my many contacts with parallel leaders over many years.

All of these materials were put together in this rather freewheeling book which attempts to bring some order to them in discussing the

[2] The Swedish government financed this survey and the U. S. Public Health Service financed the survey in the United States, including the cost of coordinating the two staffs.
[3] The specific comparison of survey results in the United States and Sweden is contained in Andersen, Smedby, and Anderson (1970).

paths taken by three health service systems in similar societies and the possibilities open to each system today.

ODIN W. ANDERSON

Chicago, Illinois
May 1972

Acknowledgments

This book would not have been possible without financial and professional support from many sources. The formulation of this book started in 1958 when I was Research Director of the Health Information Foundation, an agency established in 1950, and funded by the pharmaceutical, chemical, and drug industry for research in the organization and financing of health services. In 1962 the Foundation was invited to move to the University of Chicago as an operating unit of the Graduate School of Business, and in 1964 it was renamed the Center for Health Administration Studies. Since 1962 Grant No. HS 0080 from the National Center for Health Services Research and Development made the completion of the book possible. The concept of my book had the constant support of George Bugbee, President of the Health Information Foundation and subsequently Director of the Center for Health Administration Studies from 1962 until his retirement in 1970.

I acknowledge the early assistance of Professor Osler Peterson, Department of Preventive Medicine, Harvard University, when we traveled together on two trips in the early 1960s to interest health authorities in Sweden and Great Britain in international cooperative health systems research. In due course Professor Peterson collaborated with research teams in these two countries on in-hospital patient populations while I moved into comparative social surveys with Ronald Andersen in the United States and Björn Smedby in Sweden.

xi

In the fall of 1966 the Department of Social Medicine, Uppsala University, served as my headquarters for arranging interviews with Swedish leaders. Professor Ragnar Berfenstam, Chief of the Department, and Björn Smedby of the same department guided me in selecting people to interview and arrange appointments. Specific thanks are due Dagmar Lagerberg for her library assistance and for abstracting the journal of the Swedish Medical Association. In the fall of 1967 I carried out a parallel series of interviews in Great Britain with the Nuffield Provincial Hospitals Trust as my headquarters, counseled by Gordon McLachlan, the Director.

In the Center for Health Administration Studies special thanks are due to Joanna Kravits for gathering and organizing the statistical information in the text and appendix. She and Ronald Andersen also did a careful editing of the manuscript, as did Professor David Mechanic, Department of Sociology, University of Wisconsin.

Finally, I thank the University of Chicago and the Graduate School of Business for nurturing the institutional base required for a book like this. The book has required flexibility in timing, financing, and travel, and hence a minimum of academic bureaucracy.

O. W. A.

Contents

Tables

Charts

HEALTH CARE: CAN THERE BE EQUITY?

PART ONE

THE FRAMEWORK

I

Introduction

GENESIS OF THE BOOK

I𝔫 ᴀɴ ᴇɴᴛᴇʀᴘʀɪꜱᴇ in which there are few scientifically established criteria regarding scope, methods of organization, and general operating indicators, the question asked by those working within it and worrying about it is, How does it work elsewhere? Although characteristic of any enterprise with a paucity of scientifically determined criteria for evaluating performance—educational institutions and churches, for example—this situation is particularly common in the health services.

It is this question: "How does it work elsewhere?" which stimulated interest in investigating the development, organization, and operation of health services in other countries. The cirticisms directed at the current health services in the United States sometimes make it appear that this country has the least effective and most expensive health service system among developed countries (although the physical plant and personnel are presumed to be second to none). The ineffectiveness is usually expressed in terms of higher death rates for, say, middle-aged males dying of heart attacks and excess infant mortality in this country as compared with other industrialized countries. And the relative expensiveness is measured by the proportion of the gross national product or of national income spent for health services. The United States has relatively high mortality indices among industrialized countries and apparently the highest rank for measures of expenditures for health services. To many, this is an obvious contradiction; to others, it is a stimulus for research. This book is not intended to show that a health service in one country is "better" than that in another country—an objective that I think is not fruitful—but rather to try to indicate the context and the forces shaping the health services structure in three somewhat similar countries.

Preliminary investigations of the health services and the usual indicators of organization, expenditures, and use in the United States, Sweden, and Great Britain (hereafter referred to as England) [1] in the early 1960s revealed similarities and differences that on the surface made no sense. The usual indicators of use quoted in the literature were approximately as given in Table 1.

TABLE 1   COMPARISON OF THE UNITED STATES, SWEDEN, AND ENGLAND ON GENERALLY QUOTED UTILIZATION INDICES

Type of Use	United States	Sweden	England
General hospital admission rates per 1000 population	130	130	85
Mean length of stay	8	12	12
Number of physician visits per capita	5	3	5

These data stimulated further research, as did the fact that in the United States only about two thirds of general hospital care was paid for by insurance while in Sweden and England it was virtually free at time of service. Although there was little insurance coverage for out-of-hospital physicians' services in the United States, while physicians' services were mostly paid by insurance in Sweden and were entirely free at time of service in England, the proportions of the population seeing physicians at least once during the year were approximately the same in all three coun-

[1] The British National Health Service is divided into three separate administrative areas, England and Wales, Scotland, and Northern Ireland, each with its own budget although funded almost entirely from the Central Government and each essentially similar in structure. All statistical reporting is published according to these three administrative jurisdictions. England and Wales is, of course, by far the largest of these jurisdictions, with a population of 49,000,000 out of a total of 54,000,000 for the United Kingdom. Analytically, it does not seem worthwhile to go to the effort of combining the statistics of these three jurisdictions.

tries. Furthermore, on average there appeared to be just as many physicians' visits per person in the United States as in England, and more than in Sweden. Clearly, use of health services showed mystifying variations from country to country.

As this book will attempt to document, the health services organizations in the United States, Sweden, and England have emerged in response to certain dominant factors in their respective societies and with, so far, little directed planning in any controlled sense. Health personnel professionals may have some idea of a rational health service, but, as observed by Crozier, organizational goals stated in rational terms encounter the necessity to conform to the social systems of which the organizations are a part.[2] Incompatibilities of goals in the same social system result in trade-offs which may be rational or not, depending on the viewpoint. The optimum solution is ever elusive, because, as Crozier writes, we have to be content with the "solutions merely *satisfactory* in regard to a few particularistic criteria" of which we are aware.[3] As will be shown, there are particularistic criteria giving us fragmentary knowledge of the organization and operation of the health services.

Dissatisfaction with the current operation of the health services in all of the three countries is mounting, varying only in intensity. In great part this is because of the explicit public policy everywhere that all should have equal access to health services regardless of income or residence. This policy, then, implies some sort of directed planning to assure that facilities and personnel are in the right places in the right quantities and at least of a minimum quality. It should be quite apparent that all these considerations rely heavily on judgments as to adequacy, quality, and acceptable degree of access, but the *optimum* solution is elusive. Comprehensive planning, a concept difficult to define, appears to have this goal, but, however defined,

. . . comprehensive planning requires much creativity and originality in inventing new alternatives and adjusting old ones to new conditions and tasks; comprehensive planning requires full utilization of modern knowledge to reduce uncertainty and to deal simultaneously with a large number of variables; comprehensive planning needs highly developed tacit knowledge and intuition, to provide a feeling for the *"Gestalt"* or "configuration" of the involved situations and to apply good "subjective probabilities," based on a combination between guess and estimate, for many situations in which uncertainty cannot be reduced or contained.[4]

[2] Crozier (1964), p. 8.
[3] *Ibid.*, p. 159.
[4] Dror (1967), p. 95.

The health services in the United States, Sweden, and England form an impressionistic continuum from a loosely structured health service in the United States to a highly structured one in England, with Sweden somewhere in between. Theoretically, all countries can be placed on such a continuum, although they also share many similarities.

It would seem that the United States, Sweden, and England can be regarded as examples of Western liberal democracies characterized by autonomous interest groups, mixed economies, and representative forms of government. Brief descriptions of the dominant characteristics of the health services systems in the three countries follow to reveal what is meant by loosely and highly structured systems and to provide the reader with some idea of current characteristics.

The United States

The dominant characteristics of the organization and financing of personal health services in the United States are general hospitals owned largely by nonprofit corporations sponsored by private citizens and sectarian groups. Mental hospitals are predominantly operated by the individual states, and other long-term hospitals by an amalgamation of federal, state, and local governments. The physicians are mostly in private practice, own their equipment, and own or rent their offices. Dentists are in the same situation. Pharmacists are largely in their own retail stores, with a small proportion in hospitals.

For direct services 62 percent of the cost is paid by the private sector and 38 percent by all levels of the government. Within the private sector most of the expenditures for general hospital care but less than half the physicians' services are paid by voluntary health insurance. Other goods and services are not covered by insurance, with a few exceptions.

More than 70 percent of the population is covered by some type of health insurance written by a great variety of insurance agencies. To an increasing extent employers are contributing to the costs of health insurance. The population over 65 has government-financed insurance, that is, Medicare. Consequently, there are now many sources of funds.

Government on various levels provides care for special groups such as veterans, maternal and child health, and special diseases, such as mental illness and tuberculosis. The federal government since 1946 has given grants to the states for the construction, expansion, and renovation of general hospitals, but not in payment for services, except for special purposes and groups as mentioned.

The health services establishment is, then, relatively loosely organized, and policy decisions regarding expenditures and other matters are diffused.

Sweden

The dominant characteristic of the health services in Sweden is county and municipal government ownership of the general hospitals. These governmental units are responsible for the total cost of building, maintaining, and providing services, including specialists who are salaried members of the hospital staffs. The central government pays the general hospitals a very nominal sum *per diem* for each patient from a health insurance fund, and the counties are responsible for the rest. Enrollment in government-sponsored health insurance is mandatory for the total population.

General practitioners do not have hospital appointments but provide care outside the hospitals exclusively and make referrals to specialists on the hospital staffs. Even so, patients can go directly to specialists without first being referred. General practitioners own or rent their offices and are paid a fee for each service, and the health insurance fund refunds the patient approximately 75 percent of the physicians' charges. The general practitioners do not negotiate a fee schedule with the government but are supposed to charge according to norms established in the professional associations.

Drugs are included in the health insurance benefits, but the patient pays half the costs for prescriptions of more than 60 cents except for life-saving drugs. Pharmacists in their own retail outlets contract with the government for prescription drugs. Dental care is free to children but not to adults.

The health services system is financed from a variety of sources: payments from employers and employees; direct charges to patients; funds from county and municipal governments for general hospital care; and funds from the federal government for mental and tuberculosis hospitals. Approximately 85 percent of the funds come directly from various governmental sources or are made obligatory by government such as payroll deductions for health insurance.

England

The entire population has virtually free access to health services by signing up with a general practitioner. About 95 percent have done so.

The main characteristics of the British National Health Service can be easily described, because the central government owns and operates the entire hospital system. All services and goods are provided by the system, and almost the entire cost is paid from general tax funds collected by the central government. Only a small portion is paid by payroll deductions.

As in Sweden, the specialists are salaried members of the hospitals' medical staffs, but, unlike in Sweden, their services may not be sought directly by patients within the health insurance system. They must be referred by the general practitioners, who do not have hospital appointments. The general practitioners own or rent their own offices, but they are paid on a capitation basis arrived at by negotiations between the practitioner representatives and the government. Dental care was until recently provided at a small initial charge to patients (this charge is larger now under the aegis of the Conservative Party), and dentists are paid a fee for each service, arrived at by negotiations with the government. Prescription drugs are provided at a small charge, and pharmacists are paid according to a schedule negotiated with the government.

Thus, in contrast to the United States and Sweden, the British National Health Service is highly structured. Since it is almost entirely financed by the central government, the costs of the services are in direct competition with other obligations of the treasury. The size of the private sector is not known exactly, but it is relatively small. There are estimates that 10 to 25 percent of the population carry some limited type of private health insurance, mainly to supplement the National Health Service. In any case, over 85 percent of the funds come from governmental sources.

The health services system and methods of paying for services are "Loosest" in the United States and "tightest" in Great Britain, with Sweden occupying a position between the two countries. It can be said that the situation is more dynamic and in greater ferment in the United States than in Sweden and Great Britain because the last two countries already have a rather well defined public policy regarding the proper sharing of governmental and private responsibilities and methods of organizing and providing services. It cannot be said that the United States has yet arrived at a definite policy in this regard because even though the issue of publicly financed medical care for the aged regardless of income is now resolved, the issue has arisen for other groups.

It is, of course, possible to be even more global than my current range of countries, but the logistics of time, energy, and opportunities for wide contacts and travel set inherent limits to the number and variety of health services systems that could be encompassed. It was also felt that, unless a country was chosen outside of the Western orbit, such as the Soviet Union, adding another country would not contribute enough variability to warrant the time, energy, and resources for the purpose.

The purpose of these comparisons can be expressed in a series of intentions:

1. Attempt to formulate a framework of health services development, structure, and functioning. What elements of the system are common to all Western countries, and what are the variations?

2. Show the relationship of the structure of health services to the larger society of which it is a part—sources of funds, organizational structure, personnel, and loci of controls.

3. Relate the problem-solving styles in the health services to the problem-solving styles of the larger societies.

4. Examine possibilities for various types of planning, particularly directed planning, in each country.

Obviously, although the book is being limited to three countries, the problems discussed here will appear in any system. Ideally, problems that are solvable by some type and degree of intervention can be distinguished from those that it is illusory to assume have any optimum solution.

METHOD OF APPROACH

The assumption underlying a systems approach is that societies, institutions, and enterprises have structures and functions; otherwise they would not develop, persist, or, for that matter, die. Certainly, the persistence of an enterprise must infer some kind of structure that is persisting. This concept has a venerable history from the physical and biological sciences, has been adopted by the social and behavioral sciences, and is now enshrined in the concept of ecology, as summed up in the book by Katz and Kahn which draws on a long line of preceding theorists:

Systems theory is basically concerned with problems of relationship of structures and of interdependence rather than with the constant attributes of objects.[5]

A general systems approach is now becoming popular in the health field.[6] This gathering interest should replace the previously naive notion

[5] Katz and Kahn (1966).
[6] Anderson and Kravits (1968), Backett (1969), Hedinger (1969), Kissick (1968), May (1969), Navarro (1969), Wagner (1969). It should be noted that systems analysis as used here refers mainly to "large" systems approaches rather than to

that the health services can be manipulated piecemeal without affecting the other components of the system. The health services can be conceptualized as a system with points of entry and exit for the patient, the primary concern being with the very personal problems of disease, disability, and death. There are identifiable types of facilities and organizational structures. There are identifiable types of personnel, and there are identifiable types of medical programs, health insurance mechanisms, and training centers.

It is apparent that there is no attempt to construct a clearly delineated mathematical-type model. There is not enough appropriate information on the structure and functioning of the health services for this purpose. We are still groping to define the appropriate variables. Thus one of the purposes of this effort will be to set forth the dimensions and operations of health services from current information and on a comparative basis. It is only in recent years—say the last 15—that there has been enough information even of a structural variety about facilities, personnel, and organizational systems, not to mention indicators of use over time, to set forth the system characteristics of the health services. After doing this, there will be an attempt to formulate a "model" of the elements that make up a modern health service, the major indicators of its operation, and the assumed impact on the health levels of a population. Finally, this model will be used to show what has happened and is happening to this "model" in three countries and to generalize therefrom.

By now, it should be apparent that this comparative analysis is intended to be somewhat freewheeling. There is a contribution to be made by ranging from careful interpretations where data are available to plausible inferences where they are not. Data are available, for example, for patterns of use of health services, facilities, personnel and mortality patterns, providing a "factual universe" to draw on in describing the health services. However, when dealing with political and social philosophies and how these affect the structure and operation of the health services, the emphasis must be on plausible and reasonable inferences based on reading and experience and predilections. Inferences here are on slippery ground because there may be other interpretations that are equally plausible and reasonable. As expressed by Barrington Moore:

> All that the social historian can do is point to a contingent connection among changes in the structure of society.[7]

the "small" systems or operations research approach. A basic theoretical underpinning for the "large" systems approach is exemplified by Katz and Kahn.

[7] Moore (1966), p. 29.

This approach is justified because of the open nature of the subject, the relative paucity of data in this area, and the timeliness of presenting some kind of synthesis. The health services structure is just about ready for a detailed, rigorous, and precise systems approach to permit the testing of precise hypotheses. This book attempts to point the way to sharper conceptualization and deeper understanding by synthesizing current knowledge.

II

Elements of a Health Service

A SYSTEMS APPROACH to any enterprise requires quantifiable indicators. In this regard the health field is in a relatively primitive stage because it is not even possible to differentiate clearly between inputs and outputs. Related to this is the difficulty of how to measure "efficiency," impact of the system on health indices, and so on. Systems dealing with intangible outcomes such as health services and educational institutions in contrast to physical systems have tremendous inherent problems of conceptualization and measurement. That is, it is very difficult to demonstrate what "good" or "bad" is being done as measured by cost benefits, end results, and other economic and engineering measurements of efficiency. Human elements of satisfaction and assurance should be given relatively great weight, which has not been generally the case.

Central to the systems concept of the health services is the presence of two basic variables: the patient's perception of need for seeking service and the physician's discretionary judgment and authority to diagnose and prescribe. As long as patients and physicians require and are accorded a relatively wide range of behavior, health services organizations will necessarily remain comparatively loose in their operations. The opposite type of organization is typified by a life insurance company where decisions are based on specified and quantifiable information, such as age at death, amount of premium contributions, and the face value of the insurance policy. Discretionary judgments are not necessary.

12

In addition, as new curative or therapeutic procedures emerge, the behavior of the public toward them may be quite unpredictable. Although the chief decision maker of the allocation of health services once the patient seeks care, the physician, is by functional necessity accorded a great deal of discretionary authority to diagnose and treat as he deems appropriate, there is wide variability among physicians as to diagnostic and therapeutic procedures even when the diagnosis is specific. In their increasing attempts to rationalize and organize health services, administrators, financing agencies, and politicians become distressed and frustrated by these two "facts of life." They persist in believing that somewhere there is a Platonic medical heaven with a tidy health service. All one needs to do is to continue the search.

Because of the difficulties in the health field of defining and measuring need, demand, and discretionary judgment, discussion and debate regarding a "good" and "efficient" health services system becomes to a large extent a matter of informed opinion and experience on the part of both administrators and practitioners. This in turn leads to rather woolly administrative and political pronouncements. There are assumptions of precision and certainty which are not there. More optimistically, however, it might be said that there is more information regarding the operation of the health services than there was 20 years ago as a result of increasing research and analysis. The conceptual and empirical research literature has been proliferating to a degree that has made possible an attempt at systems conceptualization. We are still far from a systematic base of information that can guide health services research and policy short of the amount of money available.

As a beginning it is necessary to set forth the usual indicators in the health field to show means and ranges and to establish the parameters over time for the same system and currently for different systems. There are a number of such indicators now. They are the best indicators we have so far as to the operation of the health services. Although we are not always certain what they mean in terms of efficiency, performance, and so on, they do provide some reference points and a base for continued investigation. It is not necessary even to approximate the life insurance company model alluded to earlier in order to develop significant indicators for comprehending and evaluating health services systems. Our daily lives are suffused with "indicators" that give us reference points: temperature and humidity, driving speeds, baseball batting averages, prices, air pollution indices, and so on. It is useful to develop an indicators' universe in the health field as well.

A proposed schema of the elements of a health service system and the commonly used indicators are set forth below. These indicators are not necessarily exhaustive, but are inclusive enough for the purpose of this book.

AN OUTLINE OF ELEMENTS
OF A HEALTH SERVICES SYSTEM

A. Indicators of Units of Facilities

1. The general hospital is predominantly a facility for patients with short-term, acute conditions. Although seemingly precise, the definitions of short-term and acute are actually somewhat fuzzy. Arbitrary judgment declares that patients remaining in a general hospital less than 20 or sometimes 30 days are "short-term" by definition; anybody remaining longer is "long-term," and a significant minority of general hospital patients do remain longer than this.

The administrative units are usually organized according to the type of care that fits the classification of the patient—medical, surgical, obstetric, psychiatric, and emergency. Over time this kind of classification mix has changed considerably and will undoubtedly continue to do so; thus geriatric care is becoming increasingly dominant. When anesthesiology and antisepsis were first discovered and applied, the general hospital was essentially a surgically oriented institution; later, medical patients were admitted in increasing numbers; still later it became common to admit women to the hospital for deliveries; then diagnostic admissions became numerous; and so on. These classifications reveal a dynamic institution responding to external demands.

Administrative units are also determined by the type of accommodation—private, semiprivate, or ward. Whereas administrative units determined by type of care required by the patient are in great part a response to physician definition, "type of accommodation" is largely a response to social definition of proper surroundings for the patient and the extent to which amenities can be afforded. The usual Continental and Northern European pattern has been almost exclusively large and open wards (with a very small component of private rooms for the upper class), but in this country there has always been a relatively large private and semiprivate room component. Since World War II there have actually been more private and semiprivate beds in United States hospitals than ward beds. This is a function of rising standards of living resulting in changing concepts of privacy, and privacy is expensive. In Scandinavia and Great Britain there is now increasing demand for private and so-called amenity accommodations, which are supposed to be more "gracious" than ward accommodations; there has always been the presumption that the "technical quality" of patient care does not vary from one type of accommodation to the other.

Finally, administrative units are determined by the type of technical equipment and facilities required—the operating room, delivery room, pharmacy, laboratory, and x-ray department. There are others, but these are the main "ancillary services," that is, they are ancillary to the room services of "bed, board, and general nursing." Over the years, however, the ancillary services have become an increasingly larger component of the *per diem* charges, now accounting for more than one half of these charges.

Offshoots of the general hospital are outpatient and emergency departments. In the United States and Sweden, outpatient departments may serve as a first entry point for patients on their own initiative or as an entry after referral from their physician. In England, outpatient departments serve as referral agencies only. Emergency departments are supposed to serve the same purpose in all three countries, that is, as an entry point for accidents and sudden and severe illnesses. General hospitals are the only agencies that have the concentrated medical technology and appropriate staff to handle these types of patients. In reality, however, many less serious illnesses are treated in emergency rooms in all three countries.

2. In contrast to the general hospital, which is one entity, long-term hospitals and nursing homes can be divided into several distinct types.

(a) Mental hospitals. This type of hospital has historically been a separate entity from the general and acute disease hospital because the problem to society has been one of the person's behavior rather than physical illness. Behavioral problems engender a different attitude toward the "sick" person from that accorded someone who is physically ill. The philosophy of therapy is also vastly different and involves a different, much less complicated physical and technological setting. Mental hospitals have been situated out in the country, far from centers of population, in order to isolate patients. Unlike the general hospital, it is not easy to classify mental patients by type of administrative unit or by technical equipment and goods. Instead, the tendency is to make administrative classifications on the degree of freedom given patients within the hospital building and grounds or by psychiatric classification (schizophrenic, alcoholic, etc.). The recent trend has been toward psychiatric units in general hospitals for initial observation and therapy, community mental health clinics, and the minimization of institutional care. This trend represents an attempt to bring mental patients into the mainstream of medicine through the general hospital.

(b) Tuberculosis hospitals. Little need be said in describing this type of long-term hospital. For many years the demand for beds has been decreasing because of shorter lengths of stay due to chemotherapy and earlier case finding.

(c) Long-term chronic hospitals, rehabilitation facilities, and nursing homes. These facilities are regarded as providing postgeneral hospital care for patients with long-term illnesses that presumably do not require the immediate backup of full-scale medical technology usually available in a general hospital. A return to a general hospital is, of course, imminent. Nursing home facilities have been proliferating greatly during the last 10 years. They form a gray area between highly formalized health services institutions, such as the general hospital, and the home. This ambiguity is causing a great deal of administrative problems as to standards, staffing, costs, and services.

(d) Other facilities. There are other facilities that are health related but have a large "social" component, placing them on a borderline between a "health" facility and a "social" facility. Homes for the aged are a prime example, as are residential schools for the blind and deaf and for "atypical" children.

B. Indicators of Use of Facilities

This rubric refers to "events" that measure what happens in facilities. The following are the standard event units.

1. Admissions

(a) For general hospitals the admission rate is measured as the number of people per 1000 population admitted in a year's time. A refinement is the proportion of the population with one admission, two admissions, and so on in a year.

(b) For mental hospitals and tuberculosis hospitals the usual measurement is admissions per 100,000 population in a year. A refinement is the number of first admissions, second admissions, and so on.

(c) For nursing homes and other long-term chronic facilities there seems, so far, to be no standard measure of admission rates. The number of admissions per 100,000 population might well be used.

2. Length of stay and total number of days. For short-term facilities the average length of stay is regarded as a useful measure. It reveals the turnover rate of patients in a year. This type of measure is much less satisfactory for long-term institutions where many patients stay for over a year. For all types of facilities, the number of patient days per 1000 population per year is useful.

3. Expenditures. The usual gross measurement is that of total cost, but *per diem,* per case, or per bed measures, or combinations of these, are also possible. Within the facility there can be expenditure proportions by room rate (bed, board, and general nursing) and the combinations of ancillary services mentioned earlier. Cost accounting in hospitals continues to be highly judgmental as to classification.

4. Relationship to age, sex, diagnosis. All the foregoing indicators need to be related to the age, sex, and diagnosis of patients. The "case mix" of a hospital is an important factor in comparing costs with other hospitals as some diseases are much more expensive to treat than others.

For an understanding of the relationship between a facility and a community, one must also consider the education, income, residence, and so on of the prospective patient, that is, his social origin. A public goal is to "equalize" access to services regardless of income; the attainment of such a goal cannot be evaluated without knowing the access to the hospital of various income levels (standardized by age and sex, at least, and possibly also by some kind of index of illness severity).

C. Indicators of Personnel Units and Use

1. Physicians. The physician is a distinct occupational type—almost always a person with an MD degree but, in the United States, a small number of osteopaths also belong to this category. Beyond this basic criterion, however, there is great variation along several different dimensions.

(a) Site of practice. The major division here is between physicians who have their own offices and those who are hospital based. In Sweden and England there is an official difference in the practice sites. In the United States the usual pattern is for physicians to have both their own offices and admission privileges to the hospital.

(b) Specialization of medical services and the role of the general practitioner in providing patient access to this specialization. Although the types of specialists—surgeons, obstetricians, ophthalmologists, and so on—vary little between Western countries, the role of the general practitioner in relation to these specialists is very different. In the United States, the generalist usually has a hospital appointment, and it is not uncommon for the specialist to provide primary care. In contrast, in England the generalist rarely provides hospital care and the hospital-based specialist gets most patients by referral from the generalist. Sweden is somewhere in between, with generalists not usually having hospital appointments but some specialists providing primary care in a nonhospital setting.

(c) Method of reimbursement. The most common are fee for service, fee per case, capitation, and straight salary or various combinations of these. All the methods of reimbursement are self-evident except capitation. This is a method in which a physician is responsible for a known group of people and is paid a certain amount per person per year. The method of reimbursement is extremely important because of the implications it has for the organization of medical practice.

(d) Utilization of physicians' services. This is usually measured in two ways:

(1) Visits per person in a population in a year. A refinement is number of visits per person who has been a patient.

(2) Proportion of population seeing a physician in a year.

The foregoing indicators can be related to home, office, and hospital and to time of day. Another more detailed measure of utilization is type of procedure performed—preventive, diagnostic, or therapeutic. Therapeutic procedures can be divided into medical and surgical treatment, with a rough measure of the latter being surgical operations performed per 1000 population per year. These hardly exhaust the possible measures, but they are the usual gross indicators of the "doctors' job."

Finally, the number of physicians per 100,000 population or the number of people per physician gives a rough indication of potential utilization which differs over time and in different countries or sections of countries. Of course, the age, sex, diagnosis, and other "social" characteristics of patients also affect the relationship between the physician and the population he serves.

2. Nurses. The usual classification of nurses, which varies little across countries, is headed by registered nurses with their various subspecialties (public health, midwifery). There is also an intermediate category in the United States called licensed practical nurse, and a large subprofessional category called nurse's aide. The site of service is mainly but not entirely institutional—general hospitals, mental hospitals, nursing homes—but schools, physicians' offices, and industry also utilize nurses. Public health nurses provide some home care in Sweden and England. Although the percentage of physicians who are women varies greatly from country to country, there is little variation among nurses—they are overwhelmingly female.

3. Dentists. In most countries the dentist is a distinct occupational type but not as diversified by specialty as is a physician.

The site of service is almost invariably the office although there is also a small amount of hospital work done. The overwhelming majority of dentists are general practitioners, with a few limiting their practice to a specialty, usually orthodontics or oral surgery. Types of procedure performed divide roughly into preventive—checkups, tooth scaling—and therapeutic—fillings, extractions—with relatively little scope for diagnosis compared to the physician. The methods of reimbursement are similar to those for physicians, although capitation is not used.

The utilization of dentists' services is generally measured in terms of number of dental visits per 1000 population in a year or in terms of the proportion of population seeing a dentist in a year. As with the physician, age, sex, and diagnosis make for great differences here. Social factors —such as education—play an even bigger part in patient use of dentists than they do for physician use.

4. Pharmacists. The pharmacist is a distinct occupational type with a Bachelor of Pharmacy degree whose usual site of service is the retail pharmacy but who also dispenses in a hospital setting. His usual method of payment is by salary, although it is also possible for him to be paid by procedure performed (in this case each prescription filled). The prescriptions themselves can be classified as lifesaving or as less essential (a more important distinction under the British and Swedish insurance schemes than in this country), by therapeutic purpose, or by chemical components.

5. In addition to the distinct occupational types already mentioned, there are a wide range of technical supporting personnel common to the three health service systems. The most common of these are the various levels of laboratory and x-ray technologists, physical and occupational therapists and their assistants, and social workers of various types; new categories, such as that of inhalation therapist, are constantly emerging.

D. Health Level Indicators

Health services have, of course, appeared in response to disease, disability, and death. Hence the health services must handle these in such a way as to prevent, cure, manage, and rehabilitate, or at least palliate. The effect of health services per se on the patterns of disease, disability, and death is by no means clear except in easily specified conditions such as diabetes and smallpox. In any time and place there seems to be a disease and mortality pattern related to environing social and economic conditions, including health services. The "ecology" of disease is a very complicated affair. There are multiple reasons for a morbidity and mortality pattern at any given time, and not all of these reasons are amenable to modification by the health care system. Some of the principal measurements of these two indices are as follows:

1. Mortality

(a) Crude mortality rate—the number of deaths in a population per 1000 population per year.

(b) Age-specific mortality—the number of deaths in a specific age group per 1000 population in that group per year.

(c) Cause-specific mortality—number of deaths due to a given diagnosis per 1000 population in a year.

(d) Age-specific–cause–specific mortality—deaths related to age at death and diagnosis simultaneously.

(e) Survivors at given ages out of each 100,000 born alive.

(f) Curve of expectation of life—years of life remaining at given ages.

(g) Average life expectancy—other variables can of course be introduced, such as sex or race, depending on the problem to be examined.

(h) Infant mortality—the number of deaths under one year per 1000 live births in a year. Subdivisions of this are:

(1) Neonatal mortality—number of deaths within four weeks after birth per 1000 live births.

(2) Perinatal mortality—definitions vary but the primary phenomenon is viability of the fetus before and a few days after birth. Thus there may be a measurement of the number of stillbirths plus deaths under one week per 1000 live births.

These factors can be differentiated by sex, cause, number of previous births to the mother (parity), birth order, and age of mother. Neonatal mortality is largely biological in origin while postneonatal mortality has a large social component. Biological causes of mortality are much less amenable to control than those that stem from social components. This is why the greatest improvement in the mortality rate of infants has occurred between the end of the first month and the twelfth month of life.

2. Morbidity. The determination of patterns of morbidity is regarded as a more refined measure of the health status of a population than the measurement of mortality alone. Only a small proportion of illnesses result in death; thus a measure of the amount of illness can be regarded as a measure of health levels.

Other measures of health levels that by definition involve illness are number of days of illness in a year, illnesses resulting in activity limitations such as absence from work or school, or inability to engage in one's usual daily activities.

Statistics on mortality and its causes are usually routinely recorded by public agencies. Morbidity is much more difficult to measure than mortality because mortality is a discrete event whereas morbidity is open to a variety of definitions. Hence the appropriate need-demand relationship to use of services is difficult to specify. There is general agreement, for example, that a person should seek physician's care in the case of severe pain anywhere in the body, but aching muscles after unaccustomed exercise may well be expected to recover without such attention.

Great efforts are now being put forth to measure morbidity. The main methods are as follows.

(a) Household surveys asking informants about symptoms and conditions.

(b) Physical examinations of a sample of the population by a medical team.

(c) Preexisting records for reportable diseases, physicians' records, hospital records, insurance company experience, and so on.

The kinds of morbidity rates in general use follow rather closely those for mortality, that is, morbidity by age, sex, and cause, resulting in predictable patterns that vary relatively little among industrialized countries. A sticky differentiation is that between acute and chronic morbidity resulting in arbitrary definitions of duration, that is, a condition lasting less than three months is defined as acute and more than three months as chronic.

3. Other indicators. Mortality and morbidity indicators relate primarily to the "biological" status of the individual for whom health services will hopefully pay off in terms of longer life and decreased morbidity. As the survival rate from acute and short-term disease increases, there will be an increase in long-term and intractable chronic illness. Thus other indices of "payoff" need to be brought into an evaluation of the "effectiveness" of a health service. These indices involve relief of pain, relief of anxiety, measures of satisfaction, and a graceful adjustment to inevitable disabilities as a person ages. In other words, these are "quality" of life rather than "quantity" of life measures and will require a concept of payoff as yet undeveloped.

E. Financial indicators

Some financial measurements have already been alluded to, such as hospital *per diem* charges and fees. In an overall approach it is customary to break the various major components of the personal health services into the so-called "medical dollar," consisting of the following.

1. Hospital care, both short-term and long-term.
2. Physician and dental care.
3. Drugs and appliances.
4. Nursing home care.
5. Other.

Since these components are more or less autonomous, they reveal some sort of spontaneous interplay of differential expenditures for various components which intrudes into public debates. The physician is responsible for about 80 percent of the expenditures of the medical dollar, since, in addition to his own fees, he controls hospital admissions and prescribed drugs and influences the purchase of many nonprescribed drugs and appliances.

Besides the "medical dollar," other common financial measurements are percent of gross national product or gross national income, percent of family income, and percent of personal consumption spent on personal health services. Finally, another useful measure is the sources of funds for services such as government, private insurance, employer, employee, and direct payment.

THE BOUNDARIES OF THE SYSTEM

We have dealt so far chiefly with components of the health services that are "professional" and "official" both by custom and by ease of delineation. They constitute the boundaries of a relatively easily defined system with entry and exit points, hierarchies of personnel, types of patients, and so on. These components are, then, the officially and professionally recognized "helping" services regarding disease, disability, and death. Moreover, to understand the full ramifications of "health helping" services other types of practitioners should not be overlooked— chiropractors, naturopaths, faith healers—because they may well affect the functioning of the "official" system, and they certainly constitute a social expenditure. There needs to be recognition also of the role of formal supporting agencies such as those doing social service work and informal sources of support such as relatives and family members. The latter are difficult to measure, but they constitute a large reservoir of backup service for chronic invalids, despite all allegations that the family is increasingly neglecting its own.

CROSS-NATIONAL COMPARISONS

There would seem to be agreement among observers of the health facilities and personnel in Western and Northern Europe, North American, and Commonwealth countries that when one thinks of a general hospital, a physician, a dentist, a registered nurse, or a pharmacist, these facilities and occupational types are similar enough for comparison to be possible in this comparative study. The chief differences are organizational and financial, but the facilities and personnel have emerged from the same social, economic, and political developments, which in all industrialized countries resulted in autonomous professions, private and public economic sectors, and facilities shaped by the same advances in medical technology.

Sources of funding and their relative proportions in terms of the whole are exceedingly important because they represent the ultimate brake on daily operation and development for a service which has, so far, no objective limits in terms of demand, not to mention need. The usual sources of revenue, in varying proportions depending on the country, are general tax funds on both federal and local levels of government, governmental payroll deductions for this special purpose, philanthropy, voluntary health insurance, and, finally and increasingly less important, direct expenditures by patients.

III

The Liberal-Democratic Political
and Economic Matrix

IN VIEW OF THE ASSUMPTION that health services are a subsystem of the larger society, it is well to set forth the main contours of the political and economic structure that shaped them. The very fact that they emerged during the late nineteenth and early twentieth centuries while Western Europe and North America were establishing the framework for laissez faire economics and parliamentary democracy influenced their organization and structure in the respective countries. This was particularly true in determining which were private and which were governmental responsibilities and how the sources of funds were divided. This framework continues to be the matrix in which health services policies are shaped, even though the private and public sectors are less clearly delineated than they were before 1930.

It is commonly accepted among historians, political scientists, and economists that the nineteenth century witnessed the creation of the middle classes, their breakthrough to full participation in the political process, and their dominance in private enterprise.[1] Concurrently this group was the source of enterpreneurial, technical, and managerial skills, which exploited natural resources, developed the economy, and thus began to

[1] See, for example, McNeill (1963), particularly Chapter 13.

create a social surplus [2] that spilled over into other endeavors such as the arts, education, health services, and warring for national honor and expansion.[3] These social surpluses, of course, varied in amount in different countries and were allocated for various objectives and by different means.

Laissez faire in both economic development and allocation of resources and parliamentary government as a mechanism for the distribution and management of political power were assumed to promote rationality in the social process. Rationality was attained by the former through the market mechanism for goods and services in the economy and by the latter through open debate and voting in the political system. The government, through the police and the courts, was, of course, the ultimate recourse for law and order. Private activities were given free play within the umpire and law-and-order concept of the role of government.[4] The three countries used as examples in this book evolved within essentially the same liberal-democratic political and economic framework. There are naturally variations within this framework, mainly in the respective roles of the private and public sectors and their interrelationships.

A model derived from De Gré may assist in clarifying the liberal-democratic political and economic system, called the pluralistic model of mutual checks and balances in a country with more or less equal concentrations of power.[5] De Gré set forth an imaginative construct of the relationships between social structure and freedom, freedom being defined situationally rather than metaphysically: "It may be said that the amount of freedom that an individual possesses is measured by the number of thing he can do without interference from others." [6] In practice this means that

. . . freedom flourishes most when the relationships of groups are in a relative equilibrium determined by each group's having to take into account in its actions the interests, values and power of other groups. This is true according to the degree to which the various groups are relatively equal to one another, thereby insuring the improbability of any one group attaining a monopoly of control over the rest.[7]

[2] A social surplus can be defined as the surplus necessary for an economy to expand for capital investment over and above the previous level of economic growth and for health and welfare measures.
[3] Increased production has been profusely documented by Clark (1951) for many European countries and North America.
[4] Dahl and Lindblom (1953), p. 511.
[5] De Gré (1946).
[6] *Ibid.*, p. 529.
[7] *Ibid.*, p. 530.

At the one extreme of his continuum relating freedom to social structure, De Gré postulates that there is no freedom in anarchy because there
is no social structure for the individual to relate his actions to. There is
no freedom at the other end of the continuum, that is, totalitarianism,
because power is so concentrated that the individual has no group with
which to counter the state.

The pluralist model lies between these two extremes. In such a model
the social system is relatively open so that an individual or group is able
to find its niche in society in some reasonable relationship to its efforts,
ability, and aspirations within the accepted rules of the game. Inevitably,
of course, there are "winners" and "losers," and, equally inevitably, the
"losers" wish to minimize losses by sharing the resources that are produced, so as to establish an economic floor below which no individual
falls. Inevitably also there are "winners" and "losers" who win and lose
all the time, which according to Marxian theory then creates and perpetuates upper and lower classes. A pluralistic social and political system is
deficient to the extent that there are elements in society which are unable
to play in the system because of poverty, lack of education, and discrimi-
nation.

The question still remains as to what political system gives power to
the powerless as defined in the foregoing. Basically, it would seem that
unless a society subscribes to a morality that will assist the powerless even
though they are powerless, there is no help for them. To the extent that
the powerful—and in the United States it can be reasonably assumed
that 75 percent of the people have access to political power through interest groups—are unwilling to tax themselves progressively for the sake
of the lower 25 percent so that they will be able to have a reasonable
minimum, a political system can be called immoral. Ever since the emergence of the liberal-democratic-capitalistic social system, therefore, the
concept of distributive justice has been a subject of vigorous and ideological debate because, basically, it means taking from those who have and
giving to those who have not.

Early in the nineteenth century there was a prescient observation by a
Scottish clergyman, Thomas Chalmers, who was officially concerned with
the widespread poverty and pauperism of his period: "In times like the
present, the burden is not all transferred from the poor to the rich but is
shared between them; it should be a compromise between the endurance
of the one and the liberality of the other." [8] This grudging philosophy
continues. In Western countries a rapidly expanding social surplus and
concommitantly rising aspirations have enabled the sharing of this surplus as the pie became larger so that the economically comfortable group

[8] Quoted in de Schweinitz (1943), p. 110.

has not suffered an absolute deprivation but only a relatively slower rise in its standard of living. Pundits would have it that this is still a cheap way to buy off a revolution or at least a drastic shift in power.

At some indistinct point during the nineteenth century, following the American and French Revolutions and the Reform Act in Great Britain of 1832 which gave the middle classes access to parliament to counterbalance the landed aristocracy, a pluralistic social system began to develop. Smaller countries, particularly those in Scandinavia, followed suit as the franchise was expanded to the middle and working classes. The result was a tremendous increase in industrial and farm production attributable in large part to the releasing of the latent energy and talents of the middle classes.

All of these countries had by now implemented the concept of checks and balances in the political system although there was as yet limited suffrage. The United States was the first country to grant complete male suffrage to all citizens regardless of property holdings, and this was not until 1825. By 1900, Great Britain and Sweden had extended the vote to all adult men, and by 1920 all three countries had granted suffrage to women. The granting of suffrage to those groups that had previously had no political voice was an important factor in the drive for some form of distributive justice. The problems caused by the cost of illness came under consideration, and the political process became an important vehicle for social reform.

Building on De Gré's concept, it may be useful to present the liberal-democratic political and economic system as a continuum, the contours of which have remained essentially similar from the middle of the nineteenth century to the present time in all Western democracies.

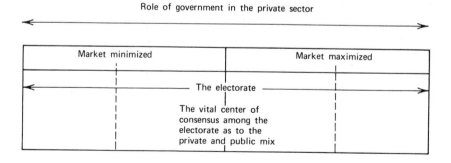

Role of government in the private sector

Market minimized	Market maximized

The electorate

The vital center of
consensus among the
electorate as to the
private and public mix

Fundamental political values constant

In this model, as depicted above, the fundamental political values remain the same over time, but the role of the government in production, distribution, and health, education, and welfare services varies between countries and, over time, within countries. Of course, this is a highly idealized construct suggested by the ideal-type methodology of Max Weber. It is a device for abstracting and conceptualizing the structure and values of systems rather than a literal description of an entire system.

In this ideal-type construct it seems reasonable to assume that some basic political values are constant, although naturally their application is a matter of degree. The breaching of these values, however, is not great enough to destroy their basic legitimacy in the political system. These values are:

1. Sovereignty of the people. Political power is legitimated by the people in an open election of candidates who in turn become the law-making body of society. The length of the term of office is limited.

2. The principle of one man–one vote. Although there has been a long struggle to approximate the ideal, the trend of enfranchisement has been clearly in this direction.

3. A judiciary independent of the executive and legislative branches of the government. In its pure form this is largely a characteristic of the American form of government; the U.S. Supreme Court can strike down a law passed by Congress when a test case is brought before it. This cannot happen in Great Britain, for example, where Parliament is supreme.

4. Flowing from the foregoing, a government of laws and not of men, that is, the consequences of given acts are predictable within the framework of law.

5. Certain fundamental rights are guaranteed: a person may not be deprived of life, liberty and property without due process of law; the right of petition and redress of grievances through the courts; and freedom of speech, assembly, and association.

Tension is inherent in all social systems, but the Western pluralistic system was revolutionary in that the government became more or less another group at interest in cooperation, competition, and negotiation with the private individual or group. Compared with previous and some contemporary societies, the individual is afforded a wide area in which to maneuver and work out his destiny in relation to others in a sense that feudal and contemporary one-party states do not purport to permit. There is, of course, serious question being raised currently as to whether the liberal-democratic pluralistic system is actually operating according to even an approximation of the theory. It would seem that this system is still operating in substance in Western countries and certainly in the three countries of major concern in this book.[9]

Referring again to the diagram depicting the "market minimized–market maximized" continuum, it is hoped that the idea of a constant set of political values providing the underpinning for the ascribed functions of private and public sectors within this continuum is clarified. What has been shifting is the "proper" mix of the private and public functions and responsibilities. Regardless of the view one has of the "proper" mix, it would seem that the minimal role of government is as follows:

1. Maintain internal order through police power.
2. Protect the country from external enemies through the military establishment.
3. Adjudicate disputes between citizens.
4. Maintain a salubrious environment which individuals could not attain by themselves.
5. Maintain education of the children up to a certain age.
6. Control the currency.
7. Provide a certain minimum subsistence for those in need.

The foregoing were the core functions to which the public sector was limited during the early stages of the evolution of the liberal-democratic-capitalistic states. Although the line separating "market minimized" from

[9] In this connection, see the sympathetic critique of liberalism by Lowi (1969). I feel the book is mistitled; it should be "The Troubles of Liberalism" or "The Agonies of Liberalism." It is quite obvious that I support the basic trends of the liberal ideology modified by the emergence of the mixed economy and the welfare state. My contemporary theorists in economics and political science are then represented by scholars such as Dahl and Lindblom, already cited. An elaboration of their thinking is contained in Dahl (1967) and Lindblom (1965). Other social scientists who have done work in this area include Blou (1964), Wildavsky (1964), and Grodzins (1966). My own book (Anderson, 1968) is pervaded by the intellectual heritage on which these authors built. It is equally obvious that I am unable to support the purity of the market concept as presented by Friedman, elegant as is the concept and its presentation.

A political-economic-philosopohical balance point for me is found in the writings of a Frenchman, Raymond Aron, as reported in the *New York Times* magazine, not to mention, of course, his books: After studying Marx, political theory, history, and theology, "I came to the conclusion that, despite their defects, parliamentary government and a mixed, Keynesian economy were the best for us. It was obvious to me that this was no ideal solution, no ideal political regime. Every system had certin negative aspects—but that, I concluded, was the essence of politics. In reaching political decisions, it was necessary to be "market maximized" is drawn through the middle of the continuum in the diagram, it can be assumed that it was farther toward the right-hand side, that is, the market-maximized extreme, during the nineteenth century than it is now. As the line moves toward the left, that is, market minimized, there is not necessarily an increase in the ownership of the means of production and distribution by the state. What has happened in what is now called "mixed" economies is the application of fiscal and monetary controls to the operation of the economy, regulation of the securities market, and related measures short of actual ownership and operation of the engines of production.[10]

Classical socialistic belief has so far stopped short of preempting the private sector as is implied by the extreme left end of the continuum. Like a quivering gauge, the line indicating the actual political situation is in some kind of undefined balance between the two extremes.

The gauge quivers because the political value constants, and the role of government in the economy, are embodied in the pervasive value of "progress," a relatively recent concept in human history. The entire "market minimized–market maximized" continuum rests on a concept of human progress, a belief that human beings through their institutions can increase and share the goods and services of life and give individuals greater and greater freedom to work out their destinies.

The difference between the two extremes of the continuum rests with the pace of change and method of change. The right end of the continuum draws on the classical economic and political theory of change through the market and limited and representative government. Such change may be fast or slow, but is nevertheless "natural" and organic, building mainly on the past. The left end of the continuum draws on the socialistic doctrines of planned economies and government programs for distributive justice and does so with "deliberate speed" and a scheduled pace. It is largely future-oriented and a historical, if not actually antihistorical. The old is corrupt; the new, and especially the unknown, utopian future is good. Finally, the right end of the extreme believes that individuals know what they want and will seek it by open competition; the just rewards go to the ambitious within the rules of the game while the weak are accorded some sort of minimum subsistence. On the left side of the continuum individuals are seen as cooperative given a socialistic structure and express this characteristic by collective efforts through the govern-

guided not by some abstract theory, but by a ratio between advantages and disadvantages." Viorst (1970), p. 35.

[10] See for example Shonfield (1969) and Dahl and Lindblom (1953).

ment. In comparison with the right extreme of the continuum, the left appears paternalistic.

Out of the foregoing balancing of beliefs has emerged the welfare state, concerned largely with mitigating and preventing destitution caused by severance from income and the labor market. The industrial revolution broke the connection between subsistence from the land and the institutionalized interdependence and mutual obligation patterns of the land tiller, landlord, and king, cemented by the church. Labor became a commodity rather than an indivisible person belonging to a class. Hence a job with money income became the source of subsistence, and jobs were increasingly owned and controlled by the emerging entrepreneurial middle class. In this context destitution was defined as a disgrace due to personal failure—with perhaps some grudging exception given to children under 5—rather than as a condition of man due to Divine Order as was assumed before the Industrial Revolution.[11]

In any case, it began to be gradually accepted that destitution results in large part from characteristics of the social system over which an individual has little control or from acts of God such as sickness and accidents rather than through deficiencies in anyone's moral qualities. The pendulum now seems to be swinging from complete individual blame toward complete societal blame for the misfortunes suffered by individuals, although the latter view continues to meet opposition.

Current concern with "incentives" in today's discussions of the inauguration of some form of a guaranteed minimum income for everybody, or a negative income tax, or whatever variant is entertained illustrates the continuation of the polar concepts of individual and social blame in the highly sophisticated form required by a complex economic system in which income is the only source of sustenance. This condition is, of course, not peculiar to Western capitalism. It inheres in industrialism itself regardless of the economic system. In Western capitalism, however, income maintenance and the sharing of risks took on a form related to individual responsibility for one's economic destiny in contrast to the collective responsibility for the individual in the communist economies. Capitalist countries have been reluctant to use general tax funds for health and welfare purposes and have been more likely to rely on specific deductions from wages and employer contributions to support health and

---

[11] This is a very brief description of an extremely complicated social, economic, and political transformation and is starkly oversimplified. The literature is vast; selected representative sources are Lippman (1937), Polanyi (1944), Schumpeter (1962), Weber (1958), Weber (1964), Wilensky (1958).

welfare developments beyond the traditional poor laws and public assistance programs.

Modern industrial society and the wage system have created five contingencies associated with the dependence on cash income:

1. Becoming unemployed—a person in the labor market has no income because of lack of a job.

2. Dying too young—a working-age person leaves survivors with no income.

3. Living too long—an old person leaves the labor market because of advanced age with no income.

4. Becoming too disabled—a person must leave the labor market either temporarily or permanently because of disability.

5. Being seriously ill—this entails costly health services and jeopardizes family financial solvency.

Before the inauguration of the official social insurance programs to cushion these contingencies, there sprang up in Western countries a great many "self-help" associations of workers, usually those in the trades, called, variously, benefit associations and friendly societies. These were voluntary organizations to which members contributed small sums periodically to help other members in case of death, unemployment, or sickness. The government regarded these associations favorably as evidence of self-reliance and prudence, qualities that kept the members off the tax-supported welfare rolls. There was also a constant but parsimonious underpinning of public assistance for the destitute as well as private charity of various kinds.

So, returning to the diagram of the "market minimized–market maximized" continuum, beginning with the latter part of the nineteenth century health and welfare philosophy was toward the right extreme of the continuum. It was assumed that individual effort through savings, life insurance, and the rudiments of voluntary health insurance would suffice even in time of need. Welfare was made exceedingly unattractive (as it is to this day) in order to discourage "excess" applications and keep taxes low.

The sharing of a social surplus is a highly volatile political issue inherent in the taxing power of the state. The horrendous descriptions of the conditions of the lower classes in Western Europe as well as in North America during the nineteenth and early twentieth centuries are usually couched in terms of an indictment of the cold-heartedness and callousness of a particular political and economic system. The existence of collective disregard for the destitute can hardly be denied, but quick imputation of motives by the critics is too facile. Such critics ignore situational circumstances of political values, economic systems, amount of social surplus, and the sheer impossibility of abolishing poverty by spreading the meager contemporary surplus more or less evenly.

It is literally only since World War II that Western democracies have been realistically able to consider abolishing poverty below a certain line because the increased productivity of modern economies is now making this a possibility. What has taken place is the sharing of a larger pie as productivity has increased so that no politically potent segment of society has suffered a net loss and most politically potent members have enjoyed a net gain. This net gain, however, has actually been a function of increased productivity and better incomes in the private sector in general rather than of redistribution of income through income taxes, social insurance, or public assistance. Poverty has thus been reduced in an absolute though perhaps not in a relative sense.[12] Whether the social surplus has been distributed equitably or not is a matter of definition and judgment and does not bear discussion here. That there has been a tremendous increase in productivity and consequent social surplus is certainly beyond dispute.

The increase in this social surplus facilitated the creation of various governmentally sponsored health and welfare measures using the ultimate power of the state to raise money in certain ways: property taxes, personal and corporate income taxes, excise taxes, taxes on goods and services, and payroll taxes. Also, of course, there was a concomitant increase in the private sector in various types of life insurance, burial insurance, sickness insurance, and health insurance. As the economy moved away from the purely private sector orientation for mitigating the five contingencies mentioned earlier, the philosophy of personal fault destitution was replaced by a philosophy of the economic system being at fault. As far as health and welfare measures were concerned, the line in the diagram dissecting the "market minimized–market maximized" areas then moved to the left. The logical result would be that all health and welfare measures would be financed by general tax funds, ideally by a progressive income tax, so that those of lower income would get more out of the health and welfare programs than they pay in taxes.

In reality, of course, the development has not been this clear-cut. Methods of financing, levels of benefits, and specification of rights to benefits have been negotiated and bargained for in the political process. The various forms legislation has taken reveal how pervasive are ideological rationalizations for methods of financing, levels of benefits, and specifica-

[12] Friedman (1963), p. 190.

tion of rights to benefits. One can hardly criticize these rationalizations unduly unless one is cynical of man's seeming inability to attack social problems directly, logically, and rationally according to some wise man's premise. What can be shown is man's ingenuity by drawing on past and current values in order to solve a problem without changing the going political and social system so much that the opposition would prevent the solution.

As health and welfare measures were inaugurated, pressured by problems created by the five contingencies mentioned, the methods of financing, levels of benefits, and specification of rights to benefits shifted from private charity and public assistance based on a family means test to social insurance and reliance on general tax funds without a means test. In this regard, as early as 1909 Winston Churchill showed his capacity for composing pungent expressions when criteria for receiving unemployment benefits were being debated. Even though the worker would contribute to the unemployment insurance fund, one member of the Royal Commission on the Poor-Law suggested he not be granted benefits if he were discharged for drunkenness. Churchill said: "I do not like mixing up moralities and mathematics." [13]

Depending on the position on the continuum the parties at interest occupied while various health and welfare measures and their financing were debated, what emerged was usually a mix of means test, specified benefits for specified rights, payroll deductions, and progressive income tax. The tendency has certainly been to regard the means-test–public-assistance approach as a residue of an increasingly expanding concept of social insurance. The word "insurance" in the liberal-democratic social welfare lexicon has been tenacious. It implies the pooling of risks—as in life and fire insurance—by premiums that are the same for everybody given the same contingency. It is embedded in self-help, self-interest, foresight, contractual relationships, and paying your own way. It does not even smack of income redistribution. Adding the warm word "social" gives the combination "social insurance" an impression both of togetherness and of actuarial realism, even though under social insurance government does rely on some degree of redistribution of income through general tax revenue and differential benefits.

An income maintenance program is quite easy to administer because all units are highly specific as to predicted cost, benefits, and eligibility. These elements can, so to speak, be spliced up into various segments; they are highly divisible. This characteristic is hardly true to the same ex-

---

[13] Gilbert (1966), p. 232.

tent for personal health services. For one thing there are two distinctly different ways of handling personal health services. They can be provided by the state, or money can be transferred to patients in the form of indemnities for incurred expenditures to help to pay the providers of health services. One concept stems from that of providing a service; the other stems from the concept of risk or contingency. It is cast in an insurance framework, and the patient "buys" from the current supply.

Returning to the "market minimized–market maximized" continuum, the more one subscribes to the extreme on the right, the more likely one is to favor private insurance, and, furthermore, profit-oriented insurance that cover certain risks such as fire, premature death, or high-cost medical episodes. As one moves toward the left of this continuum, one eventually subscribes to a completely state-owned, state-financed, and state-salaried health services system, paid for out of general tax revenues. On the right-hand side of the continuum, one is likely to believe in cash indemnity for certain contingencies and financial controls such as deductibles and coinsurance. This view regards providers of services as essentially autonomous units with which the patient deals one by one or "hires" his physician to be the manager of services. Toward the other end of the continuum one moves through a mix of various methods of delivering and financing health services to a rather monolithic structure of highly coordinated and completely governmentally financed services through general tax revenue. There would be no charge to the patient at the point of service. Any imposition of charges, however small, would be regarded as an undesirable inhibition to the use of services for early diagnosis and prevention. At the other extreme it is assumed that the patient knows his self-interest well enough not to be inhibited by small charges at time of service which can help in reducing the premium.

In short, the allocation of the social surplus for health and welfare purposes has been and continues to be an intensely debated political question. In the health field in particular this debate is becoming even more intensified as the health services continue to absorb the proliferating medical technology. The costs of health services are increasing faster than the expenditures for other goods and services in each country studied and faster than the rise in level of wages and the gross national product. Although the costs of health services have been increasing faster than the rest of the economy since 1875, an arbitrary date for the start of modern health services, since World War II there has been an acceleration that is now regarded as a "crisis."

This chapter has attempted to set forth a framework in which can be fitted the developments of the health services systems in three Western countries. It is hoped it can be shown that all the various elements mentioned within the range of the "market minimized–market maximized" continuum are present in all three countries but in varying degrees, proportions, and intensities depending on historical and contemporary factors conditioning the "mix" in each country.

PART TWO

HEALTH SERVICES AND THE LIBERAL-
DEMOCRATIC CONTEXT
IN THREE COUNTRIES

U<small>NTIL</small> <small>RECENTLY</small>, no special thought was given by authorities to the development and organization of health services. It seems that only when the basic components of modern health service had emerged and their relationships had been established did the three countries begin to think in terms of coordination, planning, and directed change. All three countries participated more or less simultaneously in the shift from an agrarian society to a pluralistic economic and political system and experienced a social surplus above subsistence needs. Consequently, by about 1920 these countries had evolved a physical plant, personnel, and organizational features that in substance remain to this day. Since then, each system has been filling out the mold. The chief shift has been in the sources of funding, both for capital investment and for day-to-day operation. This shift, from the individual to a third party, has occurred for two reasons: to protect the public from economic catastrophes caused by high-cost illness episodes and to equalize access to medical care regardless of family income.

An attempt will be made to document this sweeping statement by showing the differential developments in the three countries. This can be done (1) by country or (2) by discussing developments in all countries concurrently; both methods are used here. This book is not an exhaustive source of the details of structure and operation of the three systems. What is intended is to have the reader think about health services in large systems terms in three different contexts and to apply this knowledge to other contexts. Sufficient detail on each country is given to make it stand out as a separate entity for the reader who has a special interest in any one of the three countries. Primarily, however, this book synthesizes what happens to the elements of a modern health service in differing contexts. In that light the dominant characteristics that make health care systems differ from each other in their eventual development and the degree to which the sheer technology and occupational types of modern health services also lead to similarities are shown.

This part sets forth the dominant characteristics of society and the health services in each of the three countries before the rise of modern medicine. Modern medicine is associated with the discovery and application of rather specific medical technologies—anesthesia and antisepsis— that made wide application of surgery possible, which, in turn, laid the basis for the modern hospital during the last quarter of the nineteenth century. There were, of course, several hundred years of medical development that fed into modern medicine, extensively developed surgical procedures among them. However, the postoperative death rates from infections were unbelievably high by modern standards, not to mention the suffering that must have been caused by primitive anesthesiology.

Even before modern medicine, European countries and North America had established an extensive scatter of hospitals, largely custodial in character, as the last refuge for the destitute ill, the vagrant, the socially incompetent, and the social outcast. The problem that this variety of unfortunate people had in common was disability and illness of sufficient severity to make necessary some kind of custody.

The dominant characteristics of the three countries were certainly clear by 1900, if not before, and these will be set forth in Chapter 4. Chapter 5 shows the interacting influences of the private and public sectors as sources of funds and owners of facilities, and Chapter 6 discusses the eventual consolidation of public policy which did not really become explicit until after World War II. There is a natural chronology among the three countries regarding the accumulating influence of the public sector. This influence was felt first in Sweden, then in England, and lastly in the United States. The developmental narrative follows this chronology with, of course, inevitable overlap. Part Three discusses the performance of the health services in the three countries from 1950 to the late 1960s according to the indicators discussed in Chapter 2.

IV

The Emergence of the Dominant Characteristics

SWEDEN

Already in the second half of the eighteenth century the needs of the poor in Sweden for food, clothing, and shelter were separated from their needs for health care. This early separation of charity provided under the Poor Law and its attendant stigma from care for the sick poor had important consequences for subsequent developments. The hospital in Sweden was thus at an early date regarded as an institution for the entire community and a responsibility of the smallest unit of government, the parish. It was not saddled with the Poor Law odium of the tax-supported hospitals in the United States and both the voluntary and public hospitals in England.

Before 1800 the parishes tried to charge whenever possible, since public sources were at best meager. Because Sweden had become a strong nation-state as a result of the creation of its Baltic empire from the time of Gustavus II Adolphus (1594–1632) to the end of the Napoleonic Wars in 1815, she had a relatively well centralized government and a highly developed state bureaucratic structure necessary to run extensive military and civil enterprises.[1] Unlike England, which had a rich, powerful, and indigenous landed aristocracy, Sweden had only a small and essentially im-

---

[1] Andersson (1956), Carlsson (1961), Carlsson (1962), Rosen (1962).

39

ported landed aristocracy of "surplus nobles" from the Continent, not a sufficient counterweight to the freeholding farmers. Agriculture was the mainstay of the country and the chief source of military manpower for the frequent military forays on the European continent. Consequently, the early extensive and costly military ventures resulted in a high degree of national consciousness and control, and the Crown thought of its people's welfare in national terms.

Stimulating national development of the hospitals was the need of many returning soldiers for medical care. Venereal diseases were rampant on the European continent for years prior to the end of the Wars in 1815. The Swedish soldiers, recruited mainly from the countryside, brought their affliction home with them.

In 1818 the state levied a uniform head tax on citizens over the entire country to finance one class of hospitals called "cure-houses" that were established to care for the returning soldiers and others infected with venereal disease. One historian regarded this head tax as a kind of sickness insurance in the state's struggle against venereal disease.[2] Presumably, these "cure-houses" were scattered throughout the country in some relation to the distribution of infected soldiers. Even prior to 1818 the state had felt an increasing responsibility to subsidize the hospitals then scattered throughout the parishes. These hospitals, subsidized by the state although owned by the parishes, became known as "Crown Hospitals."

In due course, venereal disease receded, but the head tax remained as a primary source of funding for Swedish hospitals until the 1860's.[3] Nilsson, in his careful research on the history of one county, observed that financing was hardly flush; hospital care was provided "under the cold star of parsimony."[4] Even though the hospitals were meant for the entire population, the poor and the destitute were more likely to use them. Hospital services also included physicians' services. This administrative arrangement was common enough so as to be built on and solidified after 1862. Still, those who could do so turned to physicians in private practice and were treated at home.

[2] Nilsson (1966), p. 13. The chief source, however, for the early history of the Swedish hospitals is Wawrinsky (1906). This source attributes to Queen Christina a major influence in separating the Poor Law from the hospitals by her "Begger Regulation" of February 28, 1642. This regulation freed the hospitals from general care for the poor, and the hospital, according to Wawrinsky, became as translated from the Swedish an "authentic hospital," p. 9. All translations here and henceforth are by the author. Another good source is Agnell (1950).

[3] Agnell (1950), p. 31.

[4] Nilsson (1966), p. 13.

Private practice developed parallel to the tax-supported services. The state helped to support the hospital-based physicians and, as early as the late eighteenth century, the state, with the cooperation of the Swedish Academy of Medicine,[5] supported the beginning of a health officer medical corps in the counties and cities, but particularly in the outlying areas.[6] As noted earlier, there was official concern with epidemic disease, especially venereal diseases. A health officer corps was the means for attempting to control these diseases as well as for placing physicians in outlying areas. The previous military organizational experience with developing personnel and resources influenced the establishment of health officers and health departments throughout the country.[7]

The impressive state bureaucracy which Sweden had established was turned inward to develop the country after the destruction of the Swedish Baltic empire in 1815. Sweden has not directly experienced a war since that time. The evolution of the Swedish society and economy is thus a fascinating case study in the juxtaposition of adequate but not abundant resources, a talented administrative corps, a pervasive work ethic in the general population, and a liberal-democratic framework embodied in the written constitution of 1809.

This constitution was symptomatic of the changing internal distribution of political power in Western countries. Although Sweden was still far from a modern pluralistic political democracy at that time, the framework was there for the gradual enlargement of the franchise to include all adult males by 1900. Prior to 1860 there were officially four statuses—the nobility, the clergy, the middle class, and the farmers—with differential political power in the Swedish parliament. They were abolished in 1865 by an Act of Parliament, and Sweden was then on the way to a pluralistic interest group type of democracy.

The year 1862 was an important date in the evolution of the Swedish health services, particularly the general hospitals. In the continuing struggle for a share of political power and as a counterweight to the state, Sweden had been shifting toward a decentralization of administrative and political power. Up to this time the country had been divided jurisdictionally into small parishes that dealt directly with the representatives of the Crown through a score or so of units called län, each with a gover-

[5] Translation of "collegium Medicum."
[6] The chief source on the health officer corps is Björkquist and Flygare (1963).
[7] It should be pointed out that the interpretations and inferences from historical facts supplied by Swedish historians are largely the author's. Swedish historians are exceedingly factual and straightforward and it seems to be a national trait to avoid interpretations even as cautious as those in this book.

nor appointed by the Crown to handle local affairs. Although the important agrarian element had been dealt with respectfully by the Crown for generations, the farmers still did not have a strong voice in the affairs of state. They were undoubtedly joined by other elements such as the emerging middle class represented by merchants and professionals. Thus the state was moved to establish a new political unit paralleling the län.[8] Local political power was placed in elected representatives of the people in each county. The country was divided into 25 counties and four municipalities for this purpose. The County Councils in turn elected the representatives to the Upper House in a two chamber parliament, thus facilitating some checks and balances in political power.

After the counties were established as an integral part of the Swedish political system, there appeared to be some question as to what their functions would be. Up to this time the state had been subsidizing the general hospitals, even though they were owned by local parishes, and had been completely responsible for mental asylums. It was also fully responsible for the public health officers scattered throughout the country. Furthermore, the state had from the very beginning assumed responsibility, both financial and administrative, for the medical schools.

Swedish historians have not investigated why the counties were handed the responsibility for financing, maintaining, and operating the general hospitals, but the state may well have regarded this function as a local responsibility stemming from the tradition of parish responsibility which had been gradually assumed by the state through subsidies. Nilsson views the reasons as a reflection of "patriarchal conservatism, social conscience, and employer responsibility." [9] In any case, the 25 counties and four municipalities were given complete responsibility for the general hospitals and taxing power seemingly commensurate with their responsibilities.[10]

Beginning in 1864 the County Councils could receive one fifth of the retail tax on hard liquor collected by the state in the counties. According to Nilsson, the income from the liquor tax was the financial "backbone"

[8] Tingsten (1941), vol. 1, p. 13.

[9] Nilsson (1966), p. 21.

[10] In a recent report of an officially constituted government commission looking into the problem of administration and local government, or in American terms "grassroots" democracy, an interesting interpretation of why the counties were given so much responsibility for the hospitals was put forth. Recalling that the creation of the counties was really a method of distributing political power, aside from services to the people, the counties moved into a vacuum by assuming responsibilities in which other governmental units did not already have vested interests. Statens Offentliga Utredningar (47:1968), pp. 111–112.

of the newly created counties until the turn of the century,[11] supplemented by charges to patients. The latter became a decreasing source, however. Later other sources of income were tapped, such as property and personal income taxes.

Obviously, the chief political issue that the elected County Councillors had was the general hospital system, and, indeed, the expansion of the hospital was rapid: from 1861 to 1904 the number of hospitals throughout the Swedish counties and municipalities increased from 46 to 75 and the number of beds from 2960 to 7856.[12] From 1881 to 1904, a mere 23 years, expenditures more than doubled. It is certainly reasonable to infer that in 1862 neither the newly created counties nor the state could predict that the hospital and hospital-based services would eventually become such a large, expensive and important public enterprise.[13] Björkblom believes that even though the state ceased to subsidize the general hospital after the creation of the counties, its original influence gave the movement a momentum. The early influence of government, both local and central, on the hospitals and on the creation of public health officer corps laid the basis for Swedish physician services.

The private economic sector began to grow during the late nineteenth century as the physicians produced by the state-supported medical schools for whom there were no positions available in the hospitals or in public health posts turned to private practice. Hospital and public health posts were more desirable because they provided a base income. Private practice must have been economically hazardous, but even so it expanded along with the rest of the health service.

In Sweden, the public sector was initially the dominant influence on the health services. Later, this dominance was diluted by the expansion of private practice. Furthermore, within the public sector, the state lost its dominance with the delegation of the organization and financing to the counties. The hospital and the hospital-based specialists became the core of the free health service for the Swedish population accounting for the still heavy emphasis on institutional services in Sweden, and the highest bed-to-population ratio in Western countries up to the present time. The reason for the comparatively low physician-to-population ratio was possibly the centralization of financing and determination of adequate supply of physicians by the state. The Swedish Academy of Medicine had a great deal of influence on the determination of supply, since it was con-

[11] Nilsson (1966), p. 18. Nilsson told the author that in Sweden at that time the liquor tax was called "sin money."
[12] Wawrinsky (1906), p. 69.
[13] Björkblom (1942), p. 119.

sulted by the government and, of course, it was to its advantage to advise conservative estimates. Professions seem never to be generous in their estimation of adequacy when they are given a great deal of voice in determining the supply of professionals.

As the population became more affluent private medical practice became economically feasible. Moreover, by 1900 as, industry and the employed labor force grew, there arose voluntary benefit associations and insurance societies organized by the trade unions and other private groups to protect workers against various contingencies, among them loss of income through sickness absenteeism. Later private physicians' services were added and, to the degree that it was not already free, hospital care also. The state as early as the 1880's regarded these "self-help" efforts with favor and set standards of solvency, administration, and so on; these are, of course, the classic regulatory functions of government for enterprises "clothed with the public interest." [14] It was not until about 1920 that there was even the semblance of a serious political discussion for some sort of universal health insurance for physicians' services. It may well be that the relatively free hospital service for "really severe" and therefore costly illness episodes delayed serious consideration for universal health insurance for out-of-hospital services until the 1940's. Such an act was passed in 1947 and put into effect in 1955.

ENGLAND

In 1601 Elizabeth I promulgated the famous Poor Law which made the local parish responsible for the destitute. Despite this official act, hospitals originally established by the Catholic charitable orders were supported by private philanthropy from the affluent members of the new Church of England and the small, but rich, powerful, and durable aristocracy who made money from domestic estates and the expanding overseas empire. Succoring the destitute and the destitute sick was essentially a function of the aristocratic *noblesse oblige* pattern of looking after those who were on the estates or in the service of the aristocracy. Such persons lived close to a subsistence margin easily upset by illness and aging. Those who were not so fortunate as to have these connections— and there were many, because of the social transformation that society was undergoing—became the responsibility of the parishes and were supported by the meager tax rates levied for that purpose.

England, in contrast to Sweden, had a thriving aristocracy to serve as

[14] Lindeberg (1949).

the mainstay of the health and welfare establishment, such as it was: the state intervened in a very minimal sense. After 1832, when the growing middle class got the franchise and swiftly took over the reins of government with deference to the previously dominant aristocracy, the middle class was hardly anxious to raise taxes for medical care for the poor, and the *noblesse oblige* pattern persisted into the twentieth century.

Both the Swedish and the English hospitals grew out of a paternalistic [15] concept of welfare, but the Swedish concept was a product of a paternalistic state (lacking a strong aristocracy in the first place) while the English concept was a product of an aristocratic and class structured society where state intrusion was minimal and most likely not even regarded as an appropriate function.

England, being an island, developed a navy that could sail all over the world and control large land areas inhabited by people who were unable to cope with this type of Western technology. Furthermore, a naval power uses fewer resources in terms of men and materials than does a land army, such as Sweden's. English society could, then, evolve in a relatively spontaneous leisurely fashion without a central directing authority. Hospitals were not built according to any sense of equal distribution as was implicit in Sweden but according to the spontaneous initiative of members of the upper classes. England had no large armies on the Continent, and consequently few soldiers returning with venereal diseases to influence the distribution of hospital facilities. Such are the anomalies of history. England did not create a public health officer corps until the growth of cities forced attention to sanitary and environmental control after 1850. Even then these public health officers were not regarded as outposts of treatment as was true in Sweden with its far more scattered and isolated population.

In 1834 the Poor Laws were again reformed by consolidating the numerous parishes (the Elizabethan unit for the care of the destitute) into larger units under Boards of Guardians. One of the chief problems the Boards of Guardians faced was, of course, the care of the destitute sick or, in the terminology of the time, paupers. These Boards hired physicians on a competitive bid basis. This was the pattern during the greater part of the nineteenth century in England. Detailed accounts of this type of medical service [16] reveals that the physicians serving the paupers were ac-

---

[15] In an American context the word "paternalistic" is a dirty word, but it is used here as the best word in the English language to describe a type of social relationship. In a context of extreme collectivism, "individualistic" would be a dirty word.

[16] Brand (1965) and Hodgkinson (1967).

corded hardly any professional freedom by the Boards of Guardians for fear that they would exceed the budget for other than really urgent care.

By modern standards the great majority of the British population was poor. Most were regarded as the "deserving poor," who were not receiving assistance from the parish. Those receiving assistance from the parish were known as the statutory poor, or paupers. The "deserving poor" were treated at the voluntary hospitals. Abel-Smith reports that the Boards of Governors of the voluntary hospitals were made up, naturally, of members of the upper class and the aristocracy, particularly those who would assist in the financial support of the hospitals. One of the privileges of membership on these socially pretigious bodies was that the members received tickets which they could give at their discretion to poor people who could use them as an admission ticket for care in the voluntary hospitals.[17]

As the cities grew, particularly in the industrializing midlands and the north, the concentration of the population in poverty was so great that voluntary hospitals could not take on this increasing load. The cities then built municipal hospitals for statutory poor and England began to develop a two-class system of hospital care—the municipal and the voluntary hospitals. There was already present a two-class system of outpatient physicians' services implicit in the physicians hired by the Boards of Guardians and the emerging outpatient services of the voluntary hospitals. Boards of Guardians looked after the paupers and the voluntary hospitals after the "deserving poor."

Considering the affluent as well, a three-class structure of health services had developed by the end of the nineteenth century, each class being treated in separate facilities. The paupers were cared for in the municipal hospitals, the poor in voluntary hospitals, and the affluent in what the English call nursing homes, which were actually private hospitals. Most typically, however, the affluent were treated at home, since their living facilities and servants made this possible. In time, with the development of medical technology, this humane custom became impractical; all patients of whatever class needing major care had to go to the hospitals.

The medical staffing pattern of the British hospitals also reveals the class structure. Even before the advent of the modern general hospital during the second half of the nineteenth century, the Royal College of Physicians and later the Royal College of Surgeons were prestigious and powerful medical associations. As the voluntary hospitals were transformed into modern medical institutions and capitalized by the upper class, they were so heavily associated with care of the poor that it seemed

[17] Abel-Smith (1964).

natural they not be regarded as community hospitals in the Swedish and American sense, even after they became worthwhile medically for the upper classes. (Recall that the "upper class" was exceedingly small, i.e., those with any discretionary income to speak of, probably not more than 2.5 percent of the population.[18])

The voluntary hospitals became, of course, the dynamos of the medical care system, as were general hospitals everywhere, whatever the auspices. They were the primary avenues to learning medical skills leading to lucrative private practice among upper-class patients. A medical appointment to a voluntary hospital was indeed prized by a small elite of physicians, particularly in London, who felt they could make the grade because of the upper-class sponsorship. Those fortunate enough to be appointed were expected to provide free care to the charity patients and thus discharge the *noblesse oblige* duties of the hospital sponsors.

Another source of influence for the voluntary hospitals was the medical schools developed by them, further anchoring subsequent medical development to these hospitals. It was only later in the century and in the early twentieth century that municipal hospitals in association with publicly supported ("red brick") universities also began to produce physicians. It should be obvious that the English hospital system was not planned in any sense of the word. Hospitals and medical schools associated with them were the creatures of a vigorous, prosperous, and responsible upper class avoiding the power of the state and consequent taxes. London was such a powerful center of empire trade and influence that there grew up a concentration of voluntary hospitals and medical schools which the planners of health services have been unable to spread to this day.

Up to World War I the bulk of practitioners in England had no particular interest in hospital appointments. The voluntary hospital was concerned chiefly with charity patients anyway and could hardly afford the time to give free service as required. The municipal hospitals dealt mainly with the paupers—an even less desirable source of patients. So the bulk of the practitioners were competing for the paying working-class patients outside of the hospital and undoubtedly whenever possible the relatively limited supply of middle-class patients. As related by Abel-Smith, when the voluntary hospitals began to create outpatient departments for direct access, that is, patients seeking such services without referral from the general practitioner, there arose a rather serious conflict between the physicians with voluntary hospital appointments and those

[18] Cole and Postgate (1961), p. 354. Quoted from estimates made by Dudley Baxter for England and Wales in 1867.

without. Those outside did not want outpatient departments treating patients able to pay, since this would be competitive with them. The conflict was settled by the hospitals by making the outpatient departments referral services only. Thus the split came about between general practitioners and specialists which was enshrined in the structure of the National Health Service established in 1946.

Concomitantly (as in Sweden and to a comparatively limited extent in the United States), voluntary benefit associations sprang up in the industrialized cities; these were self-help associations formed by the working class, mainly by the skilled workers. The unskilled were not a part of the system. The associations were known as Friendly Societies. They were established to enable workers to handle collectively the usual feared contingencies of life which had been exacerbated by industrialization and the wage system. By the end of the century there were nearly 24,000 such benefit associations, most of them small (200 to 300 members) but a few very large (up to 700,000 members), totaling over four million members or one half the adult male population of Great Britain.[19] These associations were financed by periodic, usually weekly, contributions. The pools of money so assembled were used to assist members in distress due to death, disability, and related contingencies. In time the benefit associations also arranged for the services of general practitioners who were paid a salary, presumably related to the size of the membership. Thus was the panel practice or capitation system born, that is, attaching a known patient population to a given physician at so much per capita per year paid to the physician.

In the late nineteenth century and early in the twentieth there were reports of bargaining between the Friendly Societies and the general practitioners. The practitioners had little bargaining power because of their relatively large number, the low demand for services, and the subsistence level of th working-class population. Only a small portion of the physicians were fortunate enough to have a middle and upper-class clientele, and it is likely that such physicians were already associated with prestigious hospitals. Hence, given the circumstances, even contract practice with the Friendly Societies provided a meager but nevertheless steady income for many general practitioners. In addition, physicians could charge fees for extra services beyond the specifications in the contract and for patients not in the benefit associations.

It should be realized that while the workers were covered, their dependents were not. The emphasis was on protecting the main source of income, the wage earner. The dependents could get free service at the

[19] Gilbert (1966), p. 165.

voluntary hospitals as did the workers themselves for in-hospital services. The charity function of the voluntary hospitals for the "deserving poor" was so pervasive that no thought seems to have been given to some sort of voluntary hospital insurance until the twenties.

By the turn of the century British society had developed a health services structure with the voluntary hospitals as its backbone, although these hospitals accounted for a smaller number of beds than did the public hospitals.[20] There was a hospital-related medical staff that provided free care to the hospitalized patients and in turn earned a living from fees to private patients. These elite practitioners could treat their private patients in their homes, in nursing homes, or in the private beds provided within the voluntary hospital.

Paralleling the voluntary hospital development was the growth of the municipal hospital system. The municipal hospitals were staffed by salaried physicians and in the main served the "really poor" segment of the population. Hospitals were also built by public authorities for patients with communicable diseases and were the harbingers, according to Abel-Smith, of a government-owned hospital system.

Salient features, then, of British health services at the turn of the century were diversified sources of funding and the spontaneous development of different hospitals for different classes of society served by different segments of the medical profession. Thus the British system was made up of several segments that were more or less independent of one another reflecting the class structure. Because of the emergence of a substantial and self-conscious working class whose belief in self-help was expressed through its voluntary benefit associations, there was then an unusual amalgam in British society of self-help and *noblesse oblige*—self-help as expressed by the benefit associations and *noblesse oblige* as expressed by the voluntary hospitals. Parallel to them was a rather large, very low-income, and insecure unskilled population served by public programs.

UNITED STATES [21]

In the perspective of the period between the end of the Civil War and World War I (1865–1914) the economic, social, and political environ-

---

[20] Pinker (1966).

[21] This section and the historical material relating to the United States elsewhere in this book will in substance, unless otherwise noted, be drawn from Anderson (1968).

ment in which health services evolved in the United States was indeed an open one, little constrained by historical "barriers" that shaped the dominant characteristics of the Swedish and English cases. The American general hospital system sprang almost *de novo* out of the private-enterprise, commercial middle class. This class, in turn, sprang from a society with dominant characteristics that were not congenial to either *noblesse* or *oblige* concepts, since there was no nobility and therefore no obligation toward inferiors. The emerging *nouveau riche* had only themselves as reference points, creating the dominant business segment of American society that has been balanced by other powerful segments only since World War II. The tax-supported aspect of hospital care was a minor endeavor and apparently separate from the rapidly developing mainstream of the American hospital system as embodied in the voluntary hospital.

The voluntary hospital (like the public hospital in Sweden) was from the start a community hospital; it was designed to serve everyone and it was expected to be, in the main, self-supporting from charges to private patients.[22] Estimates made around 1900 showed that two thirds of the income for daily operations for such hospitals came from paying patients with only one third contributed from one source or another for charity patients. The nonprofit and tax-exempt status of the voluntary hospitals necessitated serving charity patients. In cities, where there were many poor people seeking care, the public facilities were hardly adequate. Furthermore, the poor provided convenient, abundant, and interesting teaching patients for the hospitals connected with medical schools. The poor were supported in the voluntary hospitals by tax funds and private philanthropy. There was also a proliferation of hospital-based outpatient departments serving the poor almost exclusively—an association that has held off the middle-class patient to this very day.

The general hospital benefitted from the surplus wealth created by the rapid development of the American economy after the Civil War and the creation of many prosperous entrepreneurs. These came from rather humble circumstances and were imbued with an ethic of hard work, financial rewards, and responsibility for worthy causes. Philanthropists typified by such names as Rockefeller, Harkness, and Johns Hopkins were major pacesetters in establishing the famous voluntary hospitals on the Eastern seaboard, and it is reasonable to infer that a similar pattern took place with less lavish, but still substantial wealth during the westward expansion of the economy. These entrepreneurs were essentially ascetic men. With few exceptions they did not know how to play with their newly acquired wealth as did maharajahs or an occasional English aristo-

[22] Corwin (1946).

crat. Life was serious; virtue was its own reward—although wealth undoubtedly helped—and the final reward among these strict Protestants was Heaven for a job well done on Earth. The natural beneficiaries for this new wealth, appearing concomitantly with medical discoveries and universal education, were hospitals, medical schools, colleges, and public libraries. Care for the poor, as such, was deemphasized among these emerging entrepreneurs and by American society in general; money for compassion had little investment potential. But money for health services and education could be regarded as an "investment" in self-help and a buttress during temporary poverty.

Thus it can be seen that the voluntary hospitals were capitalized by gifts in a breadth and depth true of no other country. A relatively small and parallel public hospital system was created by the cities for the poor. Like the English public hospitals, these hospitals were parallel to and absorbed the spillover of patients from the voluntary hospital system.

The dynamo of the health services—as was true in England and Sweden—was the general hospital, although, of course, the great bulk of health services was provided by physicians in private practice. During the late nineteenth century there were as many, and possibly even more, physicians in relation to population as there are now, and the development of the hospital naturally stimulated a scramble for hospital appointments, particularly among surgeons. Unlike the Swedish and English physicians, however, the bulk of the American physicians were able to maintain an adequate enough source of income in private practice to bargain effectively with the hospital because the growing prosperity enabled a relatively large class to buy services directly. Surgeons could provide the services for the private patient at a fee, and give free care to charity patients (from whom he learned a great deal as well) in return for a hospital appointment, and the voluntary hospital then became a viable institution.

The training of physicians took on a characteristic also typified by the social and economic context of the country in the second part of the nineteenth century.[23] The private practitioners accepted apprentices who helped them in their daily practice. In due course, many groups of physicians acquired a house or other building, set up medical schools,[24] and charged their students fees in true private enterprise fashion. These became known as "diploma mills" and were looked at askance by the emerging "respectable" medical schools associated with private and state universities after 1880 or so. With few exceptions, there

[23] Shryock (1948), Stern (1945).
[24] Flexner (1910).

was no high-quality system of medical education in the United States until after 1890. Johns Hopkins University became the pacesetter in this respect after it received several million dollars from Johns Hopkins, a railroad tycoon, to establish a university-connected medical school on the German pattern.

Before the turn of the century the medical profession was so independent—or, perhaps more accurately, regarded as having so little importance by state governments (the normal regulatory bodies)—that it was not even licensed. All a physician had to do was to hang out his shingle after having served a time with a practicing physician who determined when the novice was ready. Both the American Medical Association, founded in 1847, and the new Association of American Medical Colleges began to move in the direction of raising the standards of medical education, hence in time the standards of practice. By 1909 they had succeeded in convincing state legislators to license only physicians who were graduates of medical school certified by them, and, in short order, within a decade, the number of medical schools dropped from 135 to 66. These medical schools were affiliated with private and state universities. With westward expansion of the population, state after state established universities and professional schools—engineering, agriculture, law, education and medicine.

Thus it can be seen that by 1920 the dominant pattern of health services in the United States consisted of the voluntary hospital and private practitioners outside of the hospital, an increasing number of them having a hospital affiliation. A parallel segment of the main stream was the tax-supported city hospital, with a mixture of hospital-based and hospital-affiliated physicians and the state-supported hospitals built in association with the state university medical schools. Care for the poor was a residual of the entire system; care for the paying patient was the dominant characteristic, a characteristic that has had a powerful influence on the structure and ownership of personal health services in the United States. There were already straws in the wind of concern for the solvency of the middle-class patient in the face of rising costs. A prominent member of the American Hospital Association made the following observation at the annual meeting in 1909:

The hospitals were for the poor. They are largely now for the rich. In time they may be for all. An old question presents (sic). Has the middle class patient, who can for a term pay the family physician, a right to expect hospital treatment in time of stress?
    . . . consciously or not, all concerned in hospital management are daily

working out the beginning of this great extension—hospital provision for the Third Estate.[25]

This concern became apparent from 1915 to 1920 when 16 states introduced legislation for some form of compulsory health insurance. In the meantime, as in Sweden and England, the hospital physical plant and the health personnel had proliferated greatly, far in excess of the growth of population. All three countries now had personal health services and their structures which formed the basic matrix for subsequent developments.

[25] Brush (1909), p. 182.

V

The Mixing of the Private
and Public Sectors

BY THE TURN OF THE TWENTIETH CENTURY, all three countries had begun to
move more toward government financing and ownership of the health
services system although it was to take another 50 years before the public
policy positions of the three countries regarding the respective roles of
the private and public sectors were made explicit. In further shifts to the
public sector during this period, England led the way, followed by the
United States and Sweden.

ENGLAND

By the second part of the nineteenth century in England two voluntary
associations had appeared—the Charity Organization Society, 1869, and
the Fabian Society, 1884. The Charity Organization Society was an expression of middle-class and professional social work of the period view-
ing poverty and destitution largely as a product of personal deficiencies.
Hence two approaches were private charity and rehabilitation of the individual. Their efforts were directed mainly to the "worthy poor."

The Fabian Society was a product of the middle-class and upper-mid-
dle-class intellectuals who were socialistic in philosophy but gradualists
and nonrevolutionaries in methods for achieving such a society. In contrast to the members of the Charity Organization Society, the Fabians

viewed poverty and destitution as inherent in the system and hence worked for the transformation of society. They had faith in the application of facts and reason to the correction of social ills, working through a democratic political process: in short, democratic socialism.

Revolutionary Marxism based on violent class conflict never took hold in England for reasons that have been written about repeatedly and somewhat romantically by historians and political philosophers: the British upper-class genius for sharing political power, the counterbalancing of the middle class and the aristocracy, and the eventual absorption of the working class into the political process.[1]

The leading lights among the Fabians were Beatrice and Sidney Webb, clear products of the white-collar, professional middle classes. They were prodigious workers and published study after study of social conditions in order to influence public policy through what Beatrice Webb called "permeation" of the political parties. They had a private income and did the studies on their own time and money. Their contemporaries, Booth and Rowntree, who too carried out extensive investigations of social conditions, also had private incomes and, indeed, did the investigations themselves.

Different as the reform groups were from each other in origin and strategies for change, they were amazingly paternalistic toward the working and lower classes. Barbara Tuchman described her impression of the Webbs on the basis of extensive historical research on the period in British history from 1890 to 1914:

> They had no use for the Liberals, who understood neither the imperial nor the Socialist demands of the new age, and had little faith in a Labor Party of the untutored. What was needed was a strong party with no nonsense and a business-like understanding of national needs which would take hold of the future like a governess, slap it into clean clothes, wash its face, blow its nose, make it sit up straight at table and eat a proper diet. This could only be the conservative party, regimented by Chamberlain, advised by Mr. and Mrs. Webb, bestowing upon England the iron blessings of Tory Socialism.[2]

With increasing transfer payments from the well-to-do to the poor, it was assumed that even the meager old-age pensions, disability insurance,

---

[1] The most sophisticated sociological-economic-political-historical account known to the writer is the eminently readable book by Moore (1966), especially Chapter I, "England: the Contribution of Violence to Gradualism." Moore certainly does not replace the standard British historians such as Trevelyan; rather, he applies new social analytic tools.

[2] Barbara Tuchman (1966), Chapter 7, "Transfer of Power, England 1902–11," p. 359.

and unemployment compensation proposed might be unwisely spent. As health insurance for the working class became a political issue, there was controversy about whether the workers should be given service or provided with cash to buy the service. The conservatives and the Webbs favored a public health service with no free choice of general practitioner because the workers would not know how to select a good doctor.

The circumstances and events that led to the enactment of the National Health Insurance Act in 1911 reveal the conflict between a tax-supported public health program and a forced saving type of insurance program financed from payroll deductions. One primary source on this conflict is the Royal Commission on the Poor Laws [3] which was active from 1905 to 1909 to reexamine the total problem of welfare for the low-income segment of the population. There was great dissatisfaction in all influential quarters, social and political, with the prevailing administration of the Poor Law because destitution was not decreasing. In fact, as measured by both numbers and expenditures, it actually was increasing.[4] Furthermore, the social insurance concept was gaining some ground as an equitable method of mitigating the swings of economic fortune and was debated alongside of the increasing unpopularity of the Poor Law concept. The growing influence of the trade unions was being felt. Social insurance and health insurance became worthwhile political issues by which to use the workingman's vote.

Even before the Liberals won an overwhelming victory at the polls in 1906, the Royal Commission on the Poor Laws was constituted to look into all aspects of poverty and destitution. Beatrice Webb became a member of the Commission and contributed greatly to the amassing of data. Her mission was to scrap the Poor Laws and everything about them, particularly the means test, and to provide assistance as a right. The conservatives, on the other hand, backed by the Charities Organisation Society, sought to retain private charity and the Poor Laws as the main vehicles for helping the poor but to make them more systematic and efficient. What emerged was the classic battle between the public assistance and social insurance concepts—between the concept of the individual's being largely at fault for poverty and that of the social system's being at fault.

Organized labor had little direct political influence as yet. Labor repre-

---

[3] Royal Commission on the Poor Laws and the Relief of Distress (1909).

[4] The annual rate of pauperism in 1907 was 47.7/1000; prevalence at any given time was 22.2/1000 (Royal Commission, *ibid.*, p. 16). Pauperism increased with age, 16 percent among those 65 to 75; 28 percent, 75 to 85; and 35 percent among those 85 and over. One kind of pauper was regarded as permanent (Royal Commission, p. 23). Recall that "pauperism" at this time was really complete destitution.

sentatives were likely to work through the Liberal Party because they were not yet ready to mount their own separate party.[5] Labor was somewhat afraid of government intervention given the frequent government injunctions against strikes. Also, by 1900 the trade unions already had vested interests in their own benefit associations (Friendly Societies) and related activities, the future of which might be jeopardized by some type of government program. The main issues were the wage level and working conditions, such as the length of the workweek, rather than some form of transfer payments.

Although the Royal Commission on the Poor Laws seemed to be concerned mainly with the problem of income maintenance, there was also a great deal of interest in the medical services. The Boer War had revealed shocking health conditions among the young men recruited by the armed services, and such conditions were attributed at least in part to the status of the health services. Also, reminiscent of the contemporary United States, it was considered shameful that one of the "richest" countries in the world should have so much misery in its midst. The Report pointed to the exceedingly fragmentary nature of the health services divided by economic class, disease, varieties of sources of funds, and varieties of institutions.[6]

The Royal Commission argued against free care financed from general tax revenue. A free health service would result in high use and cost and jeopardize the existing voluntary agencies, private practice, and so on.[7]

We are of the opinion, therefore, that, while one of the first objects of a change in the present system of medical assistance should be to render it more accessible to and more readily obtainable by the working classes, it would be administered in such a way that those who contribute towards their own medical assistance (payroll deductions) should obtain it on more eligible terms than those who do not so contribute. The method should be such as not to diminish, but to encourage and stimulate a feeling of independence and self-maintenance.[8]

The differentiation between the "unworthy" and the "worthy" poor remained, although possibly in more muted form. Clearly legislation was to be "working class" and not "pauper" legislation, although the most severe medical problems were present presumably among the paupers. It was, of course, in the working class that the "swing" vote lay, to which the Liberals and Lloyd George, who became Chancellor of the Exchequer in 1908

---

[5] Pelling (1954; 1963).
[6] *Ibid.*, p. 288.
[7] *Ibid.*, p. 291.
[8] *Ibid.*

(Asquith was the Liberal Prime Minister), were to appeal in order to remain in power. What Lloyd George did was, as Dr. Thomas Jones described it, "to spike the Socialist guns with essentially conservative social measures derived from the Liberal arsenal." [9] The self-help philosophy of the majority of the members of the Royal Commission on the Poor Laws plus their continuing traditional attitude toward the poor was counterbalanced by Beatrice Webb's equally paternalistic philosophy. She wrote:

> In listening to the evidence by the C.O.S. members (Charities Organisation Society) in favor of restricting medical relief to the technically destitute, it suddenly flashed across my mind that what we had to do was to adopt the exactly contrary attitude, and make medical inspection and treatment compulsory on all sick persons—to treat illness in fact, as a public nuisance to be suppressed in the interests of the community. [10]

It is difficult to take this recommendation seriously unless one recalls that it was made at a time when public health measures to control air-, water-, and milkborne diseases were showing some effects, and, also, that atrocious hygienic habits were practiced in the working-class areas.

When Lloyd George turned his attention to health insurance in 1910 after the bulk of his social insurance program was enacted, he immediately ran into three major interests in British society who had a stake in the very principle of health insurance, not to mention methods of implementation: the Friendly Societies, the industrial insurance companies, and the British Medical Association. [11] The Friendly Societies were interested because the proposed legislation was quite directly aimed at the working-class segment of the population who were already extensively enrolled in Friendly Societies all over the country, many of which were contracting with general practitioners for their services.

The Friendly Society was essentially a conservative force rooted mainly in the nineteenth-century liberalism of self-help, and, of course, an attempt to keep clear of the Poor Laws. As Gilbert observes:

> The Societies made no appeal to the lower third of the working class. [12]

[9] Quoted in the Introduction by Sir Henry N. Bunbury in Braithwaite (1957), p. 24.
[10]. Royal Commission (1909), p. 348.
[11] The major sources for this period of agitation for health insurance are from Gilbert (1966), Braithwaite (1957), Harris (1946), and Levy (1944). Of these sources the one by Gilbert is a truly outstanding piece of historical literature.
[12] Gilbert (1966), p. 166.

The industrial insurance companies were interested because if the government were to pay undue attention to the Friendly Societies as possible administrative intermediaries between the government and the workers, this would pose a serious threat to the competitive position of the industrial insurance companies which were selling primarily funeral benefits. By 1910 the industrial insurance companies, such as Prudential, had developed an enormous market for funeral benefits by weekly door-to-door solicitation and collection, so that these agents virtually became neighborhood institutions on a personal basis. There were 30 million funeral benefit policies outstanding and 10 million new ones were sold every year.[13] Lloyd George placated the Friendly Societies first because he had a high regard for them within his liberal–laissez faire framework. He apparently gave no thought to the industrial insurance companies and the medical profession until his emerging legislative concepts became visible and subject to public debate. He ignored the medical profession, in fact, until the British Medical Association entered the political arena in full force to help shape the legislation.

Functionally, the medical profession was divided between general practitioners and hospital-affiliated specialists who engaged in private practice. The consultants and specialists who controlled the beds in the voluntary hospitals constituted the members of the Royal Colleges and were the "public" voice of the British Medical Association. They opposed the proposition that they be paid for outpatient department services to health insurance patients. There was actually little precedent for a paying working-class patient in a voluntary hospital in any event. According to Gilbert, the medical elite was concerned chiefly with keeping the "status of the 'honorary' clean," [14] that is, avoiding involvement with the government. Since the specialists would not enter into the political fray, the general practitioners were, in effect, left to fight it out alone.

The heat engendered by Lloyd George's proposed legislation is an example of pressure group politics in an increasingly pluralistic political and social system where there is a range of middle- and upper-class interests converging on a relatively simple issue—general practitioners' services for the working class (not even their dependents). Lloyd George regarded health insurance chiefly as an economic measure, not a health service measure, to keep workers out of destitution and the poorhouse, to maintain solvency, and to reduce absenteeism due to illness. He and his advisors had to bone up on the technicalities of a major piece of legislation which they learned was going to cost as much as all previous social

[13] *Ibid.,* p. 319.
[14] *Ibid.,* p. 392.

insurance legislation put together. Because of the high cost, Floyd George turned from general tax revenue to the contributory insurance concept of financing.[15]

The methods and sources of finance, the administrative agencies, and the providers of service were thrown into the political arena. The scope of benefits and the segment of the population to be benefited (except for income limits) were not at issue. The national health insurance scheme was almost naturally assumed to be working-class-oriented and to keep workers from becoming paupers. The lower third of the workers were hardly intended to be in the scheme. In this connection the words contributory and insurance bear examination. As explained by Bunbury and representatives of both prevailing Liberal and Conservative opinion, the contributory system is based on a principle that agrees with the national temperament because it entails contract and rights flowing therefrom into what they feared would otherwise become a completely governmental activity.[16]

Associated with this philosophy is the concept of insurance, which implies prudence and risk sharing.[17] General tax funds as a main source is avoided altogether, and funds are earmarked for specific purposes. According to Titmuss this issue was settled by the actuaries and the more conservative supporters of the scheme in accordance with the view that accumulating reserves for the future would be fiscally responsible and morally respectable, a clear expression of the Victorian businessman's values.[18]

Lloyd George apparently neutralized the Friendly Societies by being willing early in the discussions to use them as administrative agencies and thereby stabilize their future; the industrial insurance companies also wanted to participate in this governmental largesse and concessions were made to them in order to get the proposal enacted. Then there was the medical profession. The chief negotiating group became the general practitioners when the time came to consider method, amount, and sources of payment, scope of the working class to be covered, and the degree to which traditional professional freedoms were to be respected. The profession had not been consulted in advance at all. In anticipation, the British

[15] Braithwaite (1957), p. 71.

[16] Braithwaite (1952), Bunbury's Introduction, p. 41.

[17] In addition to the noun "insurance" itself there was the problem of the adjective to go before "insurance." The proposed legislation was at first called "invalidity insurance" which Braithwaite regarded as a "dreadful" word. Braithwaite observed that if insurance against death is life insurance, then insurance against sickness and invalidity is health insurance. This was agreed to (p. 129).

[18] Braithwaite (1957), commentary by Titmuss, p. 46.

Medical Association had gathered facts and drawn conclusions in 1911 in favor of organizing a national medical scheme based on the insurance principle, meaning contributory financing rather than general tax financing.

But Lloyd George was ahead of them and they could only react. He suppressed the emerging "revolt," as Gilbert called it, by shattering the solid front of medical opposition. The British Medical Association had set forth six conditions which reflect classic medical demands:

1. An income limit of £2 a week for the insured; no one earning more should be permitted to receive medical benefits without extra payment to the doctors.

2. Free choice of doctor by the patient, subject to the consent of the doctor.

3. Medical and voluntary benefits to be administered by the local health (later "insurance") committees, not the Friendly Societies, and all questions of medical discipline to be settled by medical committees composed entirely of doctors.

4. The methods of payment in the area of each insurance committee to be directed by the local profession.

5. Payment should be "adequate"; this was defined as a capitation fee of 8s 6d per head, per year, exclusive of the cost of medicines.

6. The profession should have adequate representation on the various administrative bodies of national health insurance.

Lloyd George readily agreed to all of these points except two with direct political implications: the income limit and the remuneration of 8s 6d. Eventually, Lloyd George worked out a compromise on the 8s 6d capitation. One concession, seemingly minor, was a lower income limit on those who would insure themselves voluntarily, that is, pay the premium themselves, thereby assuring a larger segment of the workers for private practice. Lloyd George was offering a capitation of 6s per contributor. This turned out to be apparently more than the doctors actually received from contract practice with the public at large.

The general practitioners did not go on strike, as they had threatened, and they began to sign up as private contractors with the local insurance committees set up all over the country, which in turn used the Friendly Societies and industrial insurance companies as payment agencies for the doctors who signed up. The 62 industrial insurance-approved societies had about 6.5 million members, the Friendly Societies about six million members, and the trade unions only about 500,000.[19] Premium collec-

---

[19] Gilbert (1966), p. 427.

tions started on July 15, 1912, and the medical benefits took effect on January 15, 1913, thereby building up reserves for the Friendly Societies and the industrial insurance societies.

Even this rather limited health insurance legislation was regarded as a very significant public policy breakthrough when it was enacted. Considering the tenacity of the Poor Law philosophy, the need for a shift from economic laissez faire thinking on the part of the Liberal Party regarding the role of the state in welfare, and the new experiences to be accommodated to by close to one half of the physicians in private practice, that is, the general practitioners, the National Health Insurance Act of 1911 was indeed a breakthrough. The public sector was now moving into some responsibility for physicians' services for a normally self-sustaining element of the population. The prevailing pattern of personal health services remained intact; in fact, it was stabilized into a continuing three-class level of service: (1) public hospitals and welfare doctors for the paupers; (2) general practitioner services for the workers below a certain income level and access to voluntary hospitals and/or public hospitals depending on their ability to pay something or nothing, with their dependents presumably in the same arrangement but paying the general practitioners; and (3) private practice and private beds in the voluntary hospitals, or private nursing homes, for the upper middle and upper classes. This structure remained essentially unchanged for almost 35 years.

Even though it remained intact, significant developments took place. The general hospitals were left out of the National Health Insurance Act of 1911, but difficulties of financing them both for capital needs and day-to-day costs mounted. Traditional private philanthropy was unequal to the task of doing either, not to mention both. Consequently, a larger portion of operating costs on the part of the voluntary hospitals came from paying patients, but it was never more than one half or so of costs on an average. Abel-Smith writes that by 1931 the proportion of hospital costs paid by patients had risen to 40 percent (about 10 percent before 1914), and by 1938 the proportion had gone up to 50 percent.[20] The hospitals had to make up deficits from dwindling philanthropic sources and shrinking endowments. The various voluntary hospital insurance schemes that emerged in the twenties and thirties, Hospital Contributory Associations for the working class and the Provident Associations for the middle class, could never even approximately make the voluntary hospital self-sustaining. And, of course, the public hospitals continued to carry the stigma of the Poor Laws and were shunned by both the working and the middle classes.

[20] Abel-Smith (1964), p. 385.

There was, however, official concern with both organization and finance always bubbling beneath the surface of this complex and evolving health services structure in the twenties. The operation of the National Health Insurance Act appeared to settle down after the threatened doctor revolt, and undoubtedly World War I precluded any serious consideration of tampering with the Act. In 1920, however, appeared the first Ministry of Health report, known as the Dawson report after the chairman, Lord Dawson of Penn, which set forth a highly structured and "rational" hospital and physician service system with regional hospitals, superspecialist medical centers, and less specialized satellites in the outlying areas.[21] The emphasis was clearly on a health "service" along the public health model espoused by Mrs. Webb and a few others during the debate on the National Health Insurance Act of 1911. Logically, this proposed structure was beyond debate, but undoubtedly it was too logical for the interest groups of the time, and it was not politically viable. Rather, in line with the one-step-at-a-time approach, in 1926 a Royal Commission reported on an examination of the National Health Insurance Act, the first official appraisal since the beginning of its operation 13 years previously.[22]

The main issues were the expansion of the National Health Insurance Act to include general practitioner services for the dependents of the covered workers, the inclusion of specialist services, the raising of the income limit to those of "moderate" means and the possible abolition of the approved society type of mechanism for paying the general practitioners. What resulted was a set of recommendations to change nothing at all and to commend the current operation of the Act although recognizing that it was quite limited in scope. A few members signing a minority report were in favor of expanding the services considerably, abolishing the approved society administration and moving toward a tax-supported health service.

The Commission gave an explanation which seemed to pervade the entire report for not making any substantial changes in the scope and operation of the Act:

At the same time there has come a time when the State may justifiably turn from searching its conscience to exploring its purse, and that in connexion with our present reference we are entitled to direct attention to this grave problem and to frame our recommendations in the light—or the darkness—of the economic condition of the nation.[23]

[21] Ministry of Health (1920).
[22] Royal Commission on National Health Insurance (1926).
[23] *Ibid.*

This characterizes British thinking on public financing of health services from the deliberations of the Act of 1911 to this very day.

In 1923 Parliament voted £500,000 to assist the voluntary hospitals (not the public hospitals) as a one-shot subsidy for five years. The parallel between this decision and the Hospital Survey and Construction Act of 1946 in the United States is, indeed, striking. The parallel breaks down, however, in that in Great Britain the capital subsidy was for the voluntary hospitals only, indicating their quasipublic nature as well as the political feasibility of Parliament's favoring one group of hospitals over another. Still, £500,000 spread over five years was hardly munificent even in those times; it is the intent and the symbol that are important. The grant was not renewed.

By the late thirties, then, the British health services exhibited a highly variegated pattern. Welfare medical services for the statutory poor continued through the public hospitals and the Poor Law doctor; general practitioner services for the working class through the National Health Insurance Act and approved societies were consolidated; hospital insurance for the working class through contributory schemes was growing, as were similar schemes for the middle and upper classes. According to all observers the whole structure rested on a deteriorating hospital physical plant. Private philanthropy was inadequate, assuming it ever had been adequate, and the middle classes were beginning to feel the impact of high-cost medical episodes. Public medical services or charity were not acceptable options for them. Then came World War II: "At sunset (September, 1939) the country was blacked out. Nearly six years were to pass before the evening lights were again to stream unchecked from British homes." [24]

By 1945 England was in many ways a transformed country. It had taken a major war to reorganize its health services from the welter described in the foregoing to what eventually was regarded as a unified system embodied in the National Health Service Act of 1946.

THE UNITED STATES

A few years after the enactment of National Health Insurance in England in 1911, the American Association for Labor Legislation began to look for new fields of social reform after its success in the area of workmen's compensation. It moved confidently to the next and by this time more or less self-evident social problem for the general population: how

[24] Titmuss (1950), p. 97.

to pay for the increasingly effective medical care.

As in England, the drive toward some sort of health insurance was presumed to emanate from the better paid workers and the middle class who normally were not eligible for charity. In that sense the agitation for some form of compulsory health insurance was directed to a much larger segment of the population than was ever considered in England, probably potentially as high as 60 percent, excluding the self-employed, those not attached to the labor force, and the statutory poor. Furthermore, the range of services usually considered included the general hospital and physicians' services both inside and outside of the hospitals.

The American Association for Labor Legislation drew up a model act that included hospital and physicians' services. Financing was to be tripartite: employer, employee, and the respective state governments. The model act embodied the classic insurance concept of helping people to pay for costs incurred for services.

From 1915 to 1918 there was a great deal of activity from New York to California regarding some form of universal compulsory health insurance. Ten states set up commissions to study the problem and produce some actuarial data for cost estimates, and 16 states introduced legislation. The prevailing structure of delivering services was accepted as a given, the problem being one of making health services easier to finance on the part of the general population by insurance. The American Medical Association, aware of the recent British legislation as well as that of Germany dating back to 1883, set up a Committee on Social Insurance in 1916 to study the question of health insurance in cooperation with the A.A.L.L.

The many state commissions and prevailing attitudes of "let's wait for the facts" gave an atmosphere of democracy at its rational best. As in England, however, a social reform touching a variety of vested interests immediately threw the issue of health insurance into a political arena of pressure group politics. It will be recalled that the federal government was not yet the vehicle for national concern with health and welfare problems, such responsibilities having been delegated by the Constitution to the states. Hence health insurance legislation had to be formulated state by state.

The agitation for universal and compulsory health insurance during this period was only a surface manifestation on the body politic of an uninterested public. It was not a popular political issue. The agitation seemed mainly to be a polemical battle between interest groups: the insurance companies, the drug industry, big business, and the medical profession against the A.A.L.L. and its supporters who had no big guns, not even the active support of organized labor, that is, the American Federation of Labor, representing the skilled workers at the time.

When it occurred, the backlash of the American Medical Association came as a surprise to many. A superficial appraisal of the American Medical Association activities of the period would indicate that the Association was in favor of some form of compulsory health insurance. It had supported the Committee on Social Insurance, and its editorials were sympathetic if not outrightly favorable. During this period the American Medical Association was led mainly by academically affiliated physicians whose chief concern since the turn of the century had been to improve the quality of medical education and in turn the practice of medicine. The record shows that they succeeded brilliantly. After about 1920 academicians were no longer interested in medical politics, financing and delivery systems being too complicated and remote.[25] In any case, by 1920 the state societies and the rank and file of practitioners had had an opportunity to react to the activities of the Committee on Social Insurance mainly in the person of Alexander Lambert, the outgoing president in 1920, and the chairman of the committee. "Reasonable" as the committee has been in conducting its activities and informing the membership, study was considered tantamount to espousal. At the annual meeting of the American Medical Association in New Orleans, the House of Delegates established an unambiguous official policy that stood until 1965 when the Medicare Act for the aged was passed:

Resolved, that the American Medical Association declares its opposition to the institution of any plan embodying the system of compulsory contributory insurance against illness, or any other plans of compulsory insurance which provides for medical service to be rendered contributors or other dependents, provided, controlled or regulated by any state or the Federal Government.[26]

Thus did the abortive agitation for universal and compulsory health insurance in the United States pass into oblivion.

Being unsuccessful in a frontal assault on the state legislatures, groups in favor of compulsory insurance turned to systematic study, revealing a continuing faith in the "power of facts" as the main road to social reform. Thus the Committee on the Costs of Medical Care was created in 1928, financed by six philanthropic foundations with a budget of $1,000,000, a large sum at that time solely for social research in the health field. The membership of the Committee was drawn from hospital and medical administration, law, public health, and private practice. Thus the movement toward some form of health insurance was resumed. The strategy

[25] Freyman (1965), pp. 76–80.
[26] *Journal of the American Medical Association* (1920).

was to support the movement by a rather vast factual base. These surveys were much akin to those made by Booth, Rowntree, and the Webbs in England. The goals of all these surveys were the same: the rational solution of social problems. As will be seen, the members of the Committee on the Costs of Medical Care ignored the political variables, much as their English counterparts had done. In the United States were assembled the best talents for social and health research the nation had to offer: 75 technical experts in research and statistics, generously funded and directed toward a dissection and analysis of health services expenditure, use, mortality, and morbidity on a scale never before or since exceeded.

Again, as from 1916 to 1918, there was general support for research and fact gathering; implications for action would come later. The American Medical Association editorialized, for example:

Most physicians and most economists and most social workers are willing to wait until the Committee on the Cost of Medical Care, a group with which the medical profession is cooperating wholeheartedly, has brought into the situation data on which to base reasonable action for the future.[27]

After four years of diligent work, the Committee published an impressive series of 28 reports: 27 field studies and a final report, in 1932, containing the sweeping recommendations that were supposed to flow directly from the research results. In essence, the studies—particularly No. 26 [28]—showed that illness and expenditures for health services fell unevenly over families in a year so that a small proportion experience severe illness and large medical expenditures. A few case studies were made of medical care organizations that employed physicians in group practice units attached to an industry or operated as independent plans.

Reactions to the recommendations were immediate. Majority and minority reports were prepared. The main burden of the recommendations in the majority report was, in effect, a virtual reorganization of fee-for-service and solo medical practice into group practice, plus group payment for services, that is, the insurance principle. Such a plan could be financed from either private or government sources or both.[29]

It is difficult to conceive that the supporters of the majority report really believed that both of their major recommendations could be carried out on any large scale. The insurance principle was novel enough,

[27] *Ibid.,* (1929).
[28] Falk, Klem, and Sinai (1933).
[29] Committee on the Cost of Medical Care, No. 28. The final report of the Committee on the Costs of Medical Care, adopted October 21, 1932, p. 120.

not to mention the reorganization of medical practice. Signers of the majority report, however, apparently did not believe that it was workable to attach a funding mechanism to the prevailing structure of medical practice. They surely felt that a fee-for-service method of payment was undesirable and to be eliminated as soon as possible in favor of group practice units.

The response of the signers of the minority report was as clear and unequivocal as it was vigorous. They attacked the recommendation for group practice units based in, or adjacent to, hospitals. Insurance itself was accepted in principle but cautiously. The minority felt that an insurance plan safeguarding free-choice, fee-for-service practice and under the control of the local medical society would be acceptable. The plan should be chartered as a nonprofit corporation and be open to all licensed physicians in the area.

The minority report paid no attention to one of the recommendations of the majority report, the implementation of which was to be exceedingly important in the development of health insurance in the United States. This was the recommendation that hospital insurance be provided on a voluntary basis on the part of individuals or groups in the community agreeing to pay periodic premiums for hospital care. Precedents were already appearing in Dallas, Texas, and Grinnell, Iowa.

In a famous editorial in December 1932 the American Medical Association wished to make it clear that the minority report was not to be interpreted as being opposed to any individual carrying insurance from an insurance company against the occurrence of a major illness:

Such a procedure is foresighted, American, economical. It preserves personal relationships and the free choice of physician and hospital; moreover, it makes the patient responsible to the physician and places squarely on the physician the responsibility for the care of the patient.[30]

In this same editorial, however, appeared an attack on the majority report of the C.C.M.C. which has become a classic:

The alignment is clear—on the one side the forces representing the great foundations, public health officialdom, social theory—even socialism and communism—inciting to revolution; on the other side, the organized medical profession of this country urging an orderly evaluation guided by controlled experimentation which will observe the principles that have been found through the centuries to be necessary to the sound practice of medicine.[31]

[30] *Journal of the American Medical Association* (1932), p. 1951.
[31] *Ibid.*, p. 1952.

In a short time the American Hospital Association endorsed voluntary hospital insurance as "one of the most effective ways to offset the increasing demand for more radical and potentially dangerous forms of national or state medicine." [32] Thus the American Hospital Association joined with the American Medical Association in opposition to some form of government-sponsored health insurance but took quicker and more aggressive action to carry out voluntary health insurance for hospital care.

It is difficult to determine what influence the economic depression during the thirties had on the development of voluntary health insurance. It can be assumed that an increasing number of even self-sustaining employed people were finding difficulty in paying for relatively high-cost medical care episodes. Certainly, the hospitals were experiencing reduced admissions decreasing income, and an increased charity load. Hospital insurance then became a reciprocal between the hospital's need for funds to remain solvent and the self-sustaining public's need for insurance to sustain family financial solvency.

By the mid-thirties, when the Social Security Act was being formulated, the issue of health insurance was thrown into a much larger context than ever before, beginning with the creation of the Committee on Economic Security to gather information, define the problem, and draft legislation. For the first time, then, health insurance was being considered in a national context because the problem of income maintenance for the unemployed and the retired was then regarded as a national problem, the federal government emerging as the prime source of stimulus, given its taxing power. As regards welfare, the states were paralyzed financially in any case with mounting unemployment that eventually affected 20 percent of the labor force.

The only mention of health insurance in the Social Security Bill at any stage was a recommendation that the problem be studied. Health insurance received only brief attention in the final report and recommendations of the Committee on Economic Security. The low priority given health insurance by the Committee on Economic Security gave the American Medical Association an easy victory. The striking out of "health insurance" even for study revealed the American Medical Association's intense feeling about the matter.

From 1938 to 1952, even throughout World War II, health insurance for the general population was a very live issue. In Congress there was a string of health insurance bills sponsored by Democrats. Hearings were held with the usual exchanges. No bill ever reached the floor of Congress for debate and a showdown, a significant fact revealing too narrow a base

[32] American Hospital Association (1933).

of support for a final test. The spearheads of the respective protagonists were organized labor and the American Medical Association, with ranks of less powerful supporters behind each one. Still, Congress was not moved. Preoccupation with World War II may have been one factor for its reluctance to act, but the end of the war did not change its stance. Health insurance was undoubtedly regarded as an extremely complicated and expensive measure. Concurrently, and adding to Congressional reluctance, was rapidly growing voluntary health insurance for hospital and physicians' services.

In no other country (except Canada) were the major providers of service economically strong enough and with an entrepreneurial attitude characteristic of the economy in general to mount hospital and physician insurance plans under their own auspices and control. These plans were chartered under the nonprofit corporation laws and had sufficient citizens represented on their boards of directors to be regarded as mainly acting in the "public interest." So not only did the providers shape the prevailing structure of delivering services, they also were effective in establishing a financing mechanism to assist families in paying for at least a significant proportion of high-cost episodes. The rationale was insurance, although there were endless debates on terminology: prepayment, insurance, service benefits (payment of actual charges), indemnity, and so on. The Blue Cross hospital plans and the Blue Shield medical plans grew directly out of the private, nonprofit do-it-yourself middle-class philosophy. From the beginning voluntary health insurance was an outgrowth of employed groups; and employers began to participate more and more in paying premiums as a negotiated fringe benefit in collective bargaining.

Voluntary health insurance continued to grow rapidly in an expanding war and postwar economy particularly when it was negotiated as a fringe benefit and not defined by the Wage Controls Board as an increase in wages. By 1952 voluntary health insurance covered more than half of the population and paid almost half of private expenditures for general hospital charges nationwide. It also paid about 35 percent of private expenditures for surgery. Even though enrollment was sometimes a condition of employment, hence "compulsory" in effect, the word "voluntary" persisted because the insurance was nongovernmental and the flow of funds took place in the private sector.

There was, however, political consensus on one issue: some form of federal government subsidy for the capital funding of the hospitals was needed to assure a relatively constant supply of beds. Particularly appealing was the building of hospitals in rural areas. Politically, it can be said that there were two important appeals: the rural constituency and the voluntary hospital constituency. To this end the Hospital Survey and

Construction Act (also known as the Hill-Burton Act) was passed in 1946. The agreement among the various interest groups such as the American Hospital Association and the American Medical Association was complete. This Act was the first attempt by government, state or federal, to stimulate some sort of hospital resources planning. Before states were eligible for matching grants (based on state income, population, etc.) the state had to inventory all its hospital resources and set up some criteria, loose as they were, for adding more beds to existing hospitals, building new hospitals, and renovating old ones. This program proved to be a very popular one and was developed on the precedent of federal grants-in-aid to the states. Furthermore, it was a one-grant affair for building only, obviating a continuing and presumably meddling relationship in the daily operation of the hospitals. As this program took hold, the federal government put up around 25 percent of the cost of construction, and the states and voluntary fund drives provided the large remainder. Federal funds greatly increased the provision of private funds by the kind of initial bait the subsidy represented. It is one of the prime examples of a congenial relationship between the private and public sectors in the health field.

As the balance between voluntary health insurance expansion and the potential interest in some form of government-sponsored health insurance continued, the proponents of government insurance were losing their force. This became apparent at the second national health conference which was held in 1948.

Although the deliberations of the National Health Assembly were inconclusive in affecting public policy, that is, government insurance, President Truman, who favored such insurance, was undaunted. He pressed on and three years later set up the President's Commission on the Health Needs of the Nation by means of a Congressional appropriation entitled Emergency Fund for the President, National Defense.[33] The Commission was established under the umbrella of national preparedness.

President Truman took great pains to assure the Commission complete freedom to make public policy recommendations about the health services, regardless of the known policy of the administration. To this end the President appointed an impressive commission representing the usual interest groups and representatives of the public. The competent staff, assembled quickly for the purpose, collected and organized literally all relevant information on the status of the health field up to 1950, providing a single and voluminous source of information as of that time.[34]

The reports and recommendations proved to be a benchmark not only

[33] P. L. 137, 82nd Congress, 1951.
[34] The President's Commission on the Health Needs of the Nation (1952).

of technical information but also as a mirror of emerging public policy regarding the accepted roles of private efforts and government in the United States. It is likely that new ground was broken on policy—hardly clear-cut, but the seeming stalemate revealed in the report of the National Health Assembly four years earlier was absent.

In his letter of transmittal to President Truman, the Chairman, Dr. Magnuson, crystallized the role of government in a manner never before stated so explicitly:

> The building up of our health resources in terms of training more health personnel and providing more physical facilities must start from the ground up. We have recommended Federal grants-in-aid to these and other necessary activities because we believe that the role of the Federal Government is to stimulate them, not to control them. Government must take the leadership in the promotion of good health; its major energies should go there rather than in extensive direct operation of health services.[35]

There was no consensus on means or source of finance for the health services, but for the first time there was agreement that voluntary health insurance might well be the means. There was ambiguity, an ambiguity stemming from a willingness to place all methods on fair trial. This was new. Thus it was recommended that "the present prepayment plans be expanded to provide as much health service to as many people as they can, be judged by criteria mentioned earlier . . . and be aided by government through allowing payroll deductions for government employees. . . ."[36] In the next breath there was also a recommendation to use the Social Security payroll tax mechanism to purchase health insurance for Social Security pensioners and finally that "Federal grants-in-aid be made from general tax revenue for the purpose of assisting States in making personal health services available to the general population."

The climate of discussion and debate was changing. In contrast to the "conservatives" who signed the minority report of the C.C.M.C. recommendations in 1933, it was the "liberal" members of the Commission who signed a minority report in 1952, objecting that the recommendations did not go far enough. At the end of the Truman administration, then, and beginning with Eisenhower, the first Republican President since 1932, the imminence of universal and compulsory health insurance clearly receded. A new era of public policy was at hand. De facto, voluntary health insurance was accepted as the chief vehicle for financing per-

[35] Ibid., p. vii.
[36] Ibid., Vol. I, pp. 47–48.

sonal health services for the indefinite future, and the respective roles of the private and public sectors stabilized until the early 1960s.

SWEDEN

Since Sweden already had the basic framework for a hospital service owned and operated by the counties and municipalities and since there had been official attempts to scatter physicians throughout the outlying areas in the form of practicing health officers, the most obvious immediate and emerging problem at the turn of the century was out-of-hospital physicians' services for the general population. Voluntary sickness insurance societies, largely employee-sponsored, had developed by the turn of the century, concerned chiefly with income replacement during absence from work because of illness. Slowly, these societies began to add physicians' services.

In 1910 there were as many as 2400 registered funds, and over 632,000 members or 13.4 percent of the adult population.[37] From 1910 to 1919 there were sporadic and official studies and discussions in Parliament for the possible enactment of some form of compulsory health insurance, but this movement did not seem to get going seriously until the late thirties. There never was any question that the sickness insurance Societies would be the administrative agency for a compulsory health insurance plan for physicians' services.

In 1913 a Government Commission was established to look into this question; a report was published in 1919.[38] It was proposed in principle that if health insurance was to be made compulsory, it should include the whole population rather than being limited to workers. Although it was felt that segments of the population above certain incomes should be excluded, they would be allowed to enroll voluntarily. Such insurance would include physicians' services and drugs in addition to disability insurance. Payment for physicians' services would be administered through the sickness funds. As for financing, it was suggested that two thirds be from the state from general taxes and one third be paid by the insured. In addition, it was suggested that the insured should pay one third of physicians' fees and the cost of drugs at time of service. Payment for hospital services was proposed guardedly and, if included, the sickness insurance funds were to set up controls such as on length of stay. It is unlikely, of course, that inpatient care was regarded as a serious problem

[37] Lindeberg (1949), p. 438.
[38] Ibid., p. 320.

because of the largely free service already available. The counties and municipalities were looking for other sources of income than tax funds, and compulsory health insurance could provide such a source.

The foregoing recommendations did not get formal discussion in the Swedish Parliament during the early twenties because of economic and financial considerations. Still, official concern persisted; in 1926 an expert committee was called by the government and again in 1929, but nothing came of their suggestions. Lindeberg is of the opinion that it was not until the 1930s that the Swedish sickness insurance societies had the organizational apparatus and the financial basis to take on the important problem of health insurance.[39] At this time the membership of the societies had grown to one million or about 20 percent of the adult population. Even so, only 2.5 percent of the expenditures of the sickness insurance societies were for physicians, medicines, and, to a small degree, hospitals.[40]

Although the hospital system was owned and operated by the counties and municipalities, there never seemed to be any consideration given to the possibility that these governmental units also be responsible for financing and organizing health insurance for physicians' outpatient services. Such financing was quite obviously regarded as a national problem to be implemented through the taxing power of the state. The separation of in-hospital and out-of-hospital services was very distinct, both administratively and financially.

The coming of the Social-Democratic Party to power in the middle thirties established a climate increasingly conducive to the creation of a systematic welfare state but plugged into an essentially private enterprise economy increasingly regulated by the state in its monetary and fiscal policies. This meant that for the health services there began to be serious discussions about some form of compulsory health insurance covering outpatient physicians' services or what is known in Sweden as "private practice."

Late in 1937 the Social Department of the Government was authorized to appoint a committee with the charge to review the Swedish social welfare system and make recommendations. One segment of the welfare system that received special attention was universal health insurance, and a special committee of experts and representatives of interests was set up in relation to this problem. As seems characteristic of the Swedish style, the deliberations were hardly pervaded by a sense of crisis. This was to be no crash program but a sober examination of the problems and issues, al-

[39] *Ibid.*, p. 438.
[40] *Ibid.*, p. 442.

though it seemed clear that some form of universal and compulsory health insurance would eventually be recommended. The primary issues were out-of-hospital physicians' services and drugs. It is conceivable that World War II slowed down deliberations on important public issues (the Committee did not issue a report until 1944), but government commissions in general appear to proceed with a certain logical, deliberate, and inevitable pace. This is because there are endless consultations and hearings behind the scenes with all the parties at interest so that there is little bargaining and negotiating in public, avoiding the interesting brawls witnessed routinely in the United States.

The rationale for some type of universal insurance for physicians' services were familiar and straightforward: current voluntary insurance leaves out certain low income groups, the aged, and others not attached to the labor market; it is not adequate for high-cost episodes which jeopardize family finances regardless of income; and it does little to solve the inequalities in access to the physician.[41]

The issues regarding the means to correct the foregoing problems were again straightforward, pragmatic, and nonideological. Obviously, there was an implicit ideology of insurance, risk sharing, and self-help through the state mechanism, but there were no counterideologies such as those that had made for difficulties in policy formulation in England and the United States.

By this time there were, in effect, two competing types of physician outpatient services: the polyclinics attached to the larger urban hospitals which were served by the hospital-based physicians and the physicians in private practice, with no hospital connections.[42] There was a good deal of noncontroversial discussion of expanding the polyclinics in order to provide possibly cheaper service and thereby eliminate free choice of physicians. Through a seemingly arbitrary definition of the term "insurance," it was felt that "insurance" necessitates free choice of physician, legitimates cash indemnity of patients for the costs of physicians' services incurred, and eliminates the need for a contractual relationship between the state and the participating physicians.[43] Moreover, it was felt that the subscriber should participate in paying for the insurance through payroll deduction to assure his "right" to the service.[44] The committee felt that

---

[41] *Statens Offentliga Utredningar* (15, 1944).

[42] There was, of course, a third type; the public health officers who also treated patients, but it was presumably assumed that this group would serve patients in a compulsory health insurance plan much like the private practitioners.

[43] *Statens Offentliga Utredningar* (15, 1944), p. 161.

[44] *Ibid.*, p. 119.

these psychological factors, as it called them, were important and had real consequences. The committee was acquainted with the formulations of the Beveridge Report in England which by this time was promoting a completely free service with no payment at time of service. The Swedish committee, however, was of the rather strong opinion that costs could be more easily contained by using the insurance approach rather than by a 100 percent state subsidy.[45]

The polyclinic was also discussed as a means of serving the lower income groups, the inference being that the service would be entirely free (not even a small charge at time of service); its advantage was that it could serve a great many patients. The Committee felt, however, that the practicality of free choice of physician should be tried, since it doubted that the polyclinic physician could really understand a patient's personal situation or full medical history.[46] A surprising observation in view of the utter absence of similar concern in the United States and England was that the social cost of the polyclinic might exceed its unit cost because of the waiting periods at the clinics the employed population would inevitably experience.[47]

The Committee made some reference to the attitude of the medical profession toward compulsory insurance, reporting that it was "positive" and that a cooperative relationship could be established between the physicians and the sickness insurance societies (the physician payment arm of the proposed plan).[48] The medical profession responded to impending compulsory health insurance in terms of problems of implementation rather than of principle. Apparently the principle was accepted; state intervention in health and welfare matters was hardly a controversial issue in the body politic. As revealed by the foregoing Government Report, the issue was rather one of social engineering.

As early as 1930, the Swedish Medical Association began to express opinions through its official journal. It should hardly be assumed that the Association regarded the possibility of compulsory health insurance with joy, but the principle itself did not arouse the intensity of the feelings that it did among the American and British Medical Associations, certainly not publicly. In 1930 the Board of Trustees of the Association cautioned that a universal health insurance plan for physicians' services might be inappropriate and perhaps even dangerous at this time.[49] The

---

[45] *Ibid.*, p. 117.
[46] *Ibid.*, p. 119.
[47] *Ibid.*, p. 119.
[48] *Ibid.*, p. 166.
[49] *Svenska Läkartidningen* (1930) (1).

danger was the possibility of overuse or misuse. The physicians were constantly afraid of increased pressures for service. It will be recalled that Sweden, compared to other Western countries, had appreciably fewer physicians in relation to population at this time.

Later in 1930 an utterance by the Board of Trustees of the Association accepted quite flatly the principle that compulsory health insurance is right, but it warned that measures must be taken to diminish the risks of misuse, that waiting periods (before treatment) should be long enough that all minor short-term sicknesses would be eliminated, and that specialist services should be included.[50]

The creation of the Government Committee naturally added the requisite realism to the deliberations of the Swedish Medical Association. After 1938 there continued to be concern with possible misuse of physicians' services. Harking back to the report of the previous Government Commission Report in 1919, a charge to the patient of one third of the fee at time of service was suggested. Under the proposal, outpatient specialist services were to be included; there should be no contractual arrangement between the physicians and the sickness insurance agencies paying the bills; payments for drugs should be limited to those that were lifesaving such as for diabetes; and there should be an income limit on enrollees. Even though these essentially instrumental details were proposed, there was still reluctance to endorse the principle of compulsory health insurance unequivocally. Typical questions were: Is the time opportune for such insurance? Will not "bureaucratization" of physicians' services lead to higher costs than current voluntary health insurance? Could not the state subsidize voluntary health insurance?[51]

In any event, the Swedish Parliament enacted into law the first compulsory health insurance act covering physicians' outpatient services and selected drugs in 1947. According to Swedish political protocol, however, a law is not put into effect until the government decides to do so. This was not done until 1955. The eight years were used to iron out administrative and relationship problems with the medical profession. Overlapping with the Government Commission on compulsory health insurance referred to previously was another Government Commission on physician out-of-hospital services, established in 1943 and reporting findings and recommendations in 1948, one year after the compulsory health insurance law had been enacted. This Government Commission was concerned

---

[50] *Ibid.*, (2).

[51] Sources for the foregoing are scattered throughout editorials and articles in *Svenska Läkartidningen* during the period from 1938 to 1945. Selected references are (1939), (1944), (1945).

with the contemporary structure of out-of-hospital services and their relationship to a unified and comprehensive health service. Dr. Axel Höjer, who was Director General of the National Medical Board from 1935 to 1950, caused a furor in the medical profession by advocating, in effect, a system of state medicine with salaried physicians outside of hospitals. His opinion was that salaried state medical service would enable the integration of curative and preventive services, periodic health examinations, early diagnosis, and so on.

A salaried service within the hospital did not appear to be a particular issue since it had been a standard method of payment for years. The reaction came from the physicians in full-time private practice and presumably from hospital-based physicians who also engaged in private practice on a limited basis. It should be noted at this point that hospital-based physicians had not regarded themselves as civil servants but as independent contractors analogous to university faculty. Even the local health officers had an appreciable portion of their incomes from private practice.

The recommendation for a complete salaried service came from the National Medical Board in a Government Commission Report.[52] It is of interest that the recommendation came from a government agency that had little jurisdiction over the private practitioners nor would have any in the new health insurance law which was on the statute books but which had not yet been put into effect. Under the new law, the physicians' outpatient services were to be paid for by newly constituted sickness insurance societies, 600 or so, distributed throughout the country and responsible to an insurance department in the government. These societies would pay the physicians and pharmacists and also be the distributing agents for disability benefits. What added fuel to the fire in the case of Höjer's recommendations (it seemed to be regarded as Höjer's proposal rather than as a National Medical Board proposal) was that Höjer was a declared Socialist, and even in Sweden such a label does not sit comfortably with the medical profession. Furthermore, Höjer was a career public health officer prior to his appointment rather than a clinician,[53] and the seat of power in the Swedish medical profession rested with the clinicians in the hospitals and the private practitioners, both guarding their professional prerogatives as to clinical freedom and amounts and methods of income. It was not the principle of compulsory health insurance that became the chief issue but methods and amount of

[52] *Statens Offentliga Utredningar* (14, 1948).
[53] Professor Gunnar Biörck, Department of Medicine, Serafimer Lasaretten, Stockholm, told the author in an interview that the post was offered to five clinicians, all of whom declined.

payment and professional freedom as the profession defined it. The intensity of the outburst to the Höjer proposal on the part of the profession was quite unusual, given their normally calm deliberations and discussions, indicating, of course, that an interest group has limits of tolerance. In this instance, a salaried service was beyond tolerance. Three of the five members of the Commission of which Dr. Höjer was Chairman wrote dissenting reports to the main body of the recommendations. Two representatives were medical division heads in the National Board itself, and one was the top executive officer of a County Council. Dissenting reports are unusual in Swedish Royal Commission reports because the practice is to keep discussion open until there is a consensus.

Still, the arguments put forth by the Swedish Medical Association against Höjer's recommendations were understandable, given the rather drastic changes they would entail for the contemporary pattern of practice, particularly outside of the hospitals. Sweden, like other Western countries, subscribed to incremental change, but the Swedish problem-solving style is (as compared with American and British styles) exceedingly rational, deliberate, and factual. Höjer was presumably proposing a dream. The Association took the stand that a salaried service by itself was not necessarily the best one for the country. The Association states that the continued development of the health services should be based on the current proved organization and not be bound to a detailed long-range plan. A thoroughgoing reorganization is not opportune at a time when the health services are experiencing ever-increasing demands. A completely free service [54] should not be undertaken without some experience with an expanding health insurance together with such experience with free services in other countries. Likewise, the development of preventive health services needs to be based on contemporary institutions and organizational structures. Periodic health examination of the entire population requires scientific investigations as to methods and feasibility and sufficient resources available.

When the compulsory health insurance law was put in effect in 1955, the private practitioners outside of the hospital did not have to enter into a contract with the state-controlled sickness insurance societies. Thus they guaranteed no fee schedule, and the patients paid them directly for services and were reimbursed by the local sickness insurance society for an average of three quarters of the fee for general practitioners and less in the case of specialists. The specialists in the hospitals also collected fees for outpatient services in the attached polyclinics, or in the treatment fa-

---

[54] In the Swedish context, if a patient pays a portion of the physician's charge, the service is not "free."

cilities for patients who made appointments directly, and the sickness insurance societies reimbursed the patient. The local health officers followed the same scheme. The big difference was that specialists attached to hospitals and polyclinics and health officers were paid on a negotiable fee schedule. The new act also provided partial payment for drugs.

The Swedish health services, in effect, remained quite unchanged as to structure and funding from 1862 to 1955. Voluntary health insurance evolved within the structure, mainly for outpatient physicians' services. After 1955 the primary change was in the source of payment for outpatient physicians' services and for drugs when the state began to provide help in paying for outpatient services from the physicians. The private and public sectors were becoming increasingly interrelated, but Sweden still did not have a comprehensive health service.

VI

The Consolidation of Public Policy

Iᴍᴘʟɪᴄɪᴛ ɪɴ ᴛʜᴇ sᴏᴄɪᴀʟ ᴀɴᴅ ᴘᴏʟɪᴛɪᴄᴀʟ ᴠᴀʟᴜᴇs of the three countries under study is that all people should have some kind of access to personal health services regardless of their ability to pay for them. Up to the end of World War II an adequate public policy seemed to be that of assuring some sort of minimum for the poor, usually of an emergency, last-resort, and acute nature. Even in Sweden before 1955, out-of-hospital physicians' services for the poor were provided by the Swedish public assistance programs, largely on a local basis.

The emergence of a public policy of universal and compulsory health insurance stems from the concern of the broad middle-income classes with the rising costs of medical care episodes that they find difficult to pay for out of current income or savings. Not until the politicians sensed support from the middle-income groups was universal and compulsory health insurance politically viable. The broad middle class is the vital center and, so far, the ultimate source of sanction for social reform. Not until health services had reached a certain level of incidence of costly episodes for middle-income families (for the poor, all episodes were costly almost regardless of magnitude) was there consensus that access to health services should be "equalized" for all income classes. This self-interest interpretation of the democratic-political process is reflected in the policies and events in England, Sweden, and the United States after World War II. What else is the democratic political process than the political balanc-

81

ing of self-interest groups in a matrix of basic morality to assure everyone a minimum of food, clothing, shelter—and health services? Any form of collectivism—pensions, unemployment compensation, compulsory education, and, virtually last, personal health services—has not reached the statute books until a rough majority wanted it and could sustain it. Certainly modern health care legislation can be regarded as middle-class legislation. The poor are included as a matter of course and with no deliberate attempt to compensate for their usual deprivations relative to other income classes.

The chief opponent of universal and compulsory health insurance has been the medical profession, and universal health insurance has not been achieved until the politicians have made their peace with the profession. It can be demonstrated that medicine has always been able to exact a respectable concession in terms of professional freedom to diagnose and treat, methods of payment, and even amount of payment. To the medical profession, universal coverage in its total form has always been unacceptable; some form of medical charity for the poor has always been acceptable. Universal and compulsory health insurance has been successfully enacted where the medical profession was assured some outlets—however modest—for private practice. This kind of bargaining is an integral part of the liberal-democratic heritage in all three countries.

ENGLAND

In view of the eventual opposition of the British Medical Association to details of the implementation of the National Health Service Act, it is astonishing that the Association issued as early as 1938 a program to reorganize the British health services.[1] Hardly ever has the medical profession taken the initiative in suggesting reforms before any other important body in society, particularly the government. It has usually reacted rather than acted. This is not a criticism but a description of the behavior of all professions when faced with the possibility of having to restructure their accustomed methods of practice. Eckstein is of the opinion that the

---

[1] Several books have fortunately appeared that deal quite deeply and extensively with the political maneuvering of the various groups at interest in the formulation and eventual enactment of the National Health Service. Hence it is not necessary to investigate primary sources such as the *B.M.A. Journal* and Parliamentary debates for the purpose of this book. The main secondary sources are Eckstein (1958), Forsyth (1966), Gregg (1967), Lindsey (1962), and Willcocks (1967).

B.M.A.'s proposals in 1938 were in part a response to the Socialist Medical Association's recommendations in 1933 and even to the Dawson recommendations in 1921. Eckstein believes that the B.M.A. felt the Dawson and S.M.A. proposals indulged in "medical idealizing". The purpose of the B.M.A. proposals in 1938 was to suggest something practical.[2] The Socialist Medical Association reports in particular proposed a completely rationalized, coordinated, and salaried state medical service along the classic socialist lines.

The Dawson and S.M.A. proposals contained essentially long-range objectives and few proposals for immediate action. The B.M.A., in contrast, made many short-term suggestions but came up with few long-range proposals entailing any profound changes in the organization of the health services. In brief, what the B.M.A. proposed was a tinkering with the existing structure, that is, incremental change entailing a broad extension of the contemporary health insurance act to include the entire working class, both wage earners and dependents, and a coordinated reorganization of the hospital system.

It is important that the B.M.A. felt that planned organizational change would be the major task in the next stage of health services development.[3] The B.M.A. was hardly in favor of a single unified national service, as was the S.M.A., even though it was accepting some semblance of national health planning. The B.M.A. still wished to restrict health insurance to certain income groups rather than providing it as a free service for all financed from national taxation. This was in 1938, but by 1942 the B.M.A. issued a remarkable report going far beyond the proposal of 1938.[4] This report was formulated by the Medical Planning Commission, jointly established by the B.M.A. and the Royal Colleges "to study wartime developments and their effects on the country's medical services." The commission was made up of 73 members representing virtually every viewpoint of the profession, and it is reasonable to believe that its published views were authoritative. Annual meetings of the B.M.A. following the report endorsed almost all of its more significant recommendations.

Before presenting the recommendations it may be well to return to the beginning of World War II to provide the context in which the Medical Planning Commission deliberated. Those who were adults during World War II, and particularly those who were interested in welfare and health measures "to make a better world" after the cessation of hostilities, recall the euphoria attending the publication of the Beveridge Report in 1942

[2] Eckstein, p. 117.
[3] *Ibid.,* p. 118.
[4] *British Medical Journal* (1942).

which outlined this better world.[5] Here was envisioned the end of major economic scourges of mankind—poverty, disease, and unemployment— the "archstone" of which would be a truly comprehensive health service free at time of service. At this point the tide of the war had turned after the Battle of Britain from an island and its allies being on the defensive to preparation for a massive offensive and expected victory.

In preparation for hostilities in 1939, the Ministry of Health estab- lished the Emergency Medical Service to coordinate all of the hospital fa- cilities and health personnel to take care of the wounded resulting from bombing of English cities and battle casualties from the Continent. A simple inventory and inspection of the facilities revealed the utter lack of relationship between the different parts of the system and the compara- tively sorry state of the hospitals after many years of comparative neglect for lack of capital funds.[6] There were also 100,000 persons awaiting admis- sion to voluntary hospitals, a situation that Titmuss calls "Britain's na- tional vice."

Preparation for an extreme emergency revealed the outlines of a social enterprise in stark simplicity. It may be that the gravity of the demand put on the hospital system in England exaggerated the seriousness of the condition of the hospitals. The Minister of Health ordered the consul- tants to empty beds in preparation for the expected bombings, suggesting that 100,000 beds be made ready by sending home those patients "who did not really need hospital care." The concept of need is quite elastic and, indeed, 140,000 patients were sent home and subsequent admissions were severely restricted to keep the beds empty.[7] An empty bed is, of course, a bed without income for the hospital, but the government paid the hospital a *per diem* fee for each empty bed. Thus the hospitals became accustomed to operating as a single system under the aegis of the govern- ment.

Eckstein is of the opinion that the emphasis, given the concept of a comprehensive health service in the Beveridge Report, is probably mis- placed, because it was known long before its publication that the govern- ment was seriously considering a radical reorganization of the health ser- vices after the War.[8] What is significant is that health policy was placed in the context of overall social policy regarding social services, and the government was beginning to involve itself in working out the adminis-

---

[5] Brian Abel-Smith writes, for example, in his *The Hospitals 1800–1948:* "In a sense, Britain's post-war 'Welfare State' was born in the air raid shelters, the community restaurants and the trenches" (p. 441).

[6] Titmuss (1950), p. 491.

[7] Titmuss (1950), p. 193.

[8] Eckstein, p. 134.

trative matters that Beveridge had not spelled out. Beveridge was an expert in income maintenance programs. He was also a Liberal, and his report (it was virtually his) is pervaded with an underlying philosophy of self-help and individual initiative to control one's own economic destiny, a reason why he clung to the contributory principle.[9] It might be inferred that he made personal health services an exception in that he supported an all or nothing concept both as to scope of services and universality. For example, he opposed the Medical Planning Commission's proposal (to be described more fully) that the 10 percent of the population with the highest income be left out.[10]

Beveridge certainly did not see private practice as a complement to universal health insurance. Furthermore, he apparently subscribed fully to the concept of a health service rather than the concept of an insurance risk. This led him to the belief (as it did many others) that a comprehensive health service would result in reduced disability and absenteeism:

> It is a logical corollary to the receipt of high benefits in disability (wage replacement) that the individual should recognize the duty to be well and to cooperate in all steps which may lead to diagnosis of disease in early stages when it can be prevented.[11]

This faith echoes that of the Webbs in 1910 in their attacks on piecemeal health "insurance" rather than a comprehensive health service.

The government published a White Paper on planning a health service that was derived mainly from the findings of the Emergency Medical Service Program, the Report of the Medical Planning Commission, and the Beveridge Report. There was remarkably little difference between the government White Paper and the Report of the Medical Planning Commission which had been drawn up by physicians. The Commission had paid the usual respects to positive health (which, after the war, were enshrined in the objectives of the World Health Organisation) and had recommended as the fundamental objective that everyone should somehow have access with a minimum of barriers to all health services—general practitioners, specialists, hospitals and other institutions, and home care —that might be needed. To achieve this ambitious objective, the Commission had assumed three minimal conditions:

1. Central planning of health services by public authority.
2. The organization of general practice in health centers, and the organization of hospitals on a regional basis.

[9] Beveridge, pp. 6–7.
[10] *Ibid.*, p. 160.
[11] Beveridge, p. 158.

3. Within this framework there should be preserved the patient's free choice of physician (presumably general practitioners), the voluntary hospital system should be maintained, and there should be some way for the medical profession to be represented in the administrative structure.

Some important issues were left for negotiation: method of paying physicians (although a salaried service was greatly opposed); the proportion of the population to be covered, an income limit being implicit; and how the system was to be financed—by general tax funds, contributions from employers and employees, or both. What is astonishing is that the Commission subscribed unequivocally to a unified, centrally planned health service based on a reorganized arrangement for general practice, a regionalized hospital service, and ultimate governmental control of some kind either through the Ministry or a medical "corporation." The latter already had precedents in other enterprises such as the British Broadcasting Corporation.

From an American perspective, the foregoing recommendations by physicians seem unbelievable unless the attitudes and activities are seen in the perspective of British social history and political structure. In the British political system generally there has been a deep respect for the central government. Crown, Parliament, Civil Service—these represent the elite agents of British society. On the other hand, there has been little respect for local government, particularly among the medical profession. To have local government run the health services was hardly palatable to the general practitioners, not to mention the specialists. What the profession seemed to feel in its jousting with third-party payers was the normal professional desire to maintain its autonomy as to freedom to diagnose and treat, and a voice in the administration of the medical enterprise. The profession therefore initially fought the inclusion of Friendly Societies as intermediaries in the administration of the Health Insurance Act of 1911 but was mollified by representation on the Local Insurance Committees. This is the chief reason why the profession has consistently fought a salaried service. The profession seems to feel that they can drive their best bargain with the central government and be free of possibly petty entanglements with local officials and administrators.

In any case, in the euphoria of the World War II emergency when Britain was as united as it had ever been, and the prospect of the implementation of the thoroughgoing recommendations of the Medical Planning Commission was still somewhat distant and theoretical, it was possible for the profession to submerge its immediate short-range fears and think in global terms. But the government was also thinking in global terms, and in 1943 with the publication of the White Paper the profession was faced with the immediate political realities of a plan in which they had already shown their hand.

As Eckstein summarizes so well:

> The profession was caught in an unenviable dilemma. It favored medical reform; it opposed, by reason and instinct, the intrusion of nonmedical organizations into medical affairs; but there could be no medical reform without such intrusion. There is very little in the professions's behavior after 1942 which makes sense without an understanding of this dilemma and the B.M.A.'s consequent wavering between the need for change and the dreadful implications of change.[12]

Thus the principles on which the White Paper [13] was based had become generally accepted by 1944, even by the B.M.A. Comprehensiveness of the services to be offered the public was a given. There would be free choice of physician and the maintenance of the traditional physician-patient relationship. Furthermore, the profession would be given a substantial influence in the administrative aspects of the scheme, with administration areas set up especially for the health services, that is, not attached to a local governmental unit but forming a national system culminating in the Ministry of Health.

Willcocks neatly delineates three primary interests which had to be dealt with and which had varying degrees of political leverage.[14]

1. Those with skills, chiefly of course the physicians.
2. Those with administrative positions—the existing administrators of municipal hospitals and local public health activities.
3. And those with property, that is, the voluntary hospitals, with prestige and influence out of proportion to their number.

As for those with skills, the White Paper was directed explicitly to general practitioners and only implicitly to specialists. All general practitioners who chose to practice in the system (there was no compulsion to do so) were to contract with a central organization; this agency, composed mainly of physicians themselves, would also be concerned with the distribution of general practitioners by so-called negative control in overdoctored areas. If a physician chose to practice in a health center rather than his own private office, he would come under the jurisdiction of local authorities (a sure way, incidentally, of discouraging the development of

[12] Eckstein, p. 132.
[13] Ministry of Health (1944).
[14] Willcocks (1967).

health centers). Physicians could choose freely between health centers and private practice in their own offices and be paid by salary and capitation respectively. A fee-for-service concept of payment with the government footing the bill appears to have been unthinkable in the British concept. Ostensibly, this feeling is based on the fear of lack of control of units of service, but a deeper reason is the repugnance of British social values to a fiduciary relationship between the helper and the helped, except possibly among those of equal rank in the upper classes. The White Paper also made some reference to the possibility of compensating general practitioners for the loss of goodwill associated with their practices. It was very common for retiring physicians to sell their practice to younger physicians; this possibility of sale was regarded as a return on capital investment.

The White Paper made no reference to specialists, as such. Their adequacy and proper distribution was assured to the hospital authorities; physicians in voluntary hospitals were to be paid for their services to ensure proper distribution as was already being done in municipal hospitals. The specialists were to be appointed through appropriate machinery, but further details were postponed until the publication of the Ministry of Health Report of the Inter-Departmental Committee on Medical Schools in 1944. There would be special services provided by local government such as clinic services, home nursing, health visiting, and school health. No provisions were suggested at this point for dental and optical services.

The financial underpinning was very simple and in line with equalitarian distributive principles. All services were to be free of charge at point of service to anyone who sought them. No patient or physician, however, was forced to use the service.

Private practice was permissible, although hardly facilitated and encouraged. The private sector was not regarded in social strategic terms as an adjunct or as a complement to the public sector; it has been accepted grudgingly, even more grudgingly than the public sector is accepted in the United States. British thinking to this day, except for a few economists, somehow does not regard the public and private sectors as complementary alternatives. The private sector is at best a necessary evil to accommodate some physicians and patients who wish to be outside of the system. The service was to be financed out of general taxation and local taxation, and possibly partially out of contributory insurance. Clearly a general tax system was in substance envisioned.[15]

15 The cost was estimated by the White Paper as £130 million. Beveridge had estimated £170 million. There is no necessary discrepancy in these estimates because of varying assumptions of scope, public and private funding, and so on.

Parliament accepted the White Paper enthusiastically. Eckstein observes that "the only sour notes of a session which was otherwise all sweetness and light were struck by certain spokesmen of the medical Left who thought the proposals were not sufficiently unequivocal in their commitment to a free national service, and a few spokesmen of the medical Right who were worried about the implications rather than the actual proposals of the scheme." [16] The White Paper clearly enjoyed a wide acceptance, and the Ministry of Health began to negotiate with the parties at interest as to the specific elements of legislation.

The government rather quickly eliminated the bargaining power of local governments and the voluntary hospitals after the White Paper. It was hardly a fierce struggle. The entire tenor of the previous proposals from various quarters gave short shrift to local government as the source of organization, administration, and public accountability. Local public health departments and the city health officers who administered the municipal hospitals had too low a prestige to be able to embrace the voluntary hospital and its physicians.

The local health authorities retained control of the traditional public health activities—maternal and child health programs, public health nurses, nurse-midwives, home visiting—and took on the additional responsibility of such health centers for general practitioners as would be built. These activities were to be funded by local taxation and subsidies from the central government in somewhat equal proportions. This then became one of the tripartite segments of the National Health Service, that is, the Local Health Councils' responsibility to the locally elected officials. It is an example of the influence of the past on the structure of the National Health Service. Presumably the local health councils would not give up their traditional activities; the physicians and the voluntary hospitals did not want to be a part of them; nor did the physicians and voluntary hospitals care to bother with public health activities even if they could control them. Despite the global concept of a "national health service" the eventual structuring of the service was a rather direct response to the interests of clinically oriented physicians, that is, diagnosis and treatment and not case-finding and prevention. Public-health-oriented professionals are frequently critical of the heavy clinical orientation of the National Health Service, but that the Service did take this form is hardly surprising. Cure and pain relief have always been more dramatic than the more subtle and delayed rewards of prevention.

As for those with property, it was by no means certain that the hospitals would become nationalized, particularly the voluntary hospitals, dur-

---

[16] Eckstein, p. 139.

ing the early period of the negotiations between the hospitals and the government. It does not appear either that the voluntary hospitals were unalterably opposed to nationalization, but it seems that the concept itself was a new one in British political history. Somewhat parallel to American history, the British government was more likely to buy health services for its nonpoor, that is, the workers in the case of the National Health Insurance Act of 1911, than to take on the services themselves. The consensus was that the voluntary hospitals could not raise needed capital funds because of years of neglect of their physical plant and destruction from bombing.[17] It seemed only natural to have the government take over the whole responsibility rather than indulge in subsidies for capital financing and contracts for services. After the voluntary hospitals agreed to be nationalized, they obviously lost their source of bargaining power. The implications were stupendous because this agreement enabled a regionalization of the British hospital system by fiat. Still as a reflection of relative levels of power and prestige, the teaching hospitals with medical schools, chiefly in London and associated with the Royal College of Physicians and Surgeons, were regarded as a special enclave of hospitals directly responsible to the Ministry of Health and independent of the regional boards which were set up for the other hospitals. The teaching hospitals maintained that they were islands of excellence and also relatively high-cost and therefore should not be amalgamated with the other hospitals. The specialists in these hospitals were thus given more direct access to the Ministry of Health than were other specialists.

The next, and most formidable, interest group was the physicians. When this profession met a concrete proposal head on, even though it resembled in substance that of the Medical Planning Commission mentioned previously, it fell back on familiar defense lines as to professional prerogatives, values, and amounts and methods of payment. Sources of payment were negotiable, but the bargaining centered on terms which the profession everywhere in liberal-democratic societies believed nonnegotiable in principle: nonsalaried service, a strong voice on policy-making and administrative bodies, free choice of physician, and no interference with the prerogatives of diagnosis and treatment. Their position was that professional service should be controlled by the profession within the constraints only of the total budget that society sees fit to appropriate, and here also the profession should have maximum influence. Furthermore, as in the case of the British situation, the profession wanted no truck with local government; the general practitioners in this connection did not want health centers which implied a salaried service for them.

[17] See, for example, Titmuss, p. 72.

Finally, the profession wanted the right to engage in private practice.

The government in substance met these demands, a victory for the profession. The Act still entailed continuing negotiations with the profession on the terms of the Service within that framework. Indeed, the profession was increasingly restive up to 1948 near the inauguration of the National Health Service, and two plebiscites taken by it showed a majority in opposition. The opposition was not to the concept of a free service (a dilemma the profession was constantly getting into because it is difficult to separate a principle from the implications for its implementation) but to continued fear of a salaried service, particularly after the Labour government replaced the wartime coalition government in 1945.

There are, of course, many reasons for the softening of opposition on the part of the medical profession, other than possibly the primary one of the specialists coming "to the aid of the Service" in Eckstein's words. In a society where the rule of law is so central and where it has been legitimized by the deliberations of elected representatives of the people, it borders on anarchy for an affected group to refuse cooperation. In the last analysis a legislative body must act and not be dictated to by a minority on the substance of the legislation.

Another reason why the opposition of the British profession weakened was that the existing National Health Insurance Act of 1911 would expire automatically on the appointed day, thereby depriving general practitioners of income from their past patients should they refuse to contract with the new Service. Moreover, the government had arranged to buy the goodwill that general practitioners felt they had in their practices only if they joined the new Service within a specified time. These were rather heady conditions on which to test one's principles.

In essence, then, the general practitioners carried on their accustomed arrangements, that is, panel practice and capitation payments, but expanded them to include the entire population; and the specialists were paid salaries for services they had normally provided gratis before the enactment of the National Health Service. By contemporary standards these were good salaries plus, in effect, tenure and rather unquestioned professional freedom to diagnose and treat as they deemed appropriate. The latter was no less true, really, for general practitioners, although they were subject to possible disciplinary action by the Local Executive Councils handling their contracts.

The consultants also gained on another peculiarly British point. To reward the consultants over and above their regular salaries for special clinical, research, and other professional contributions, a Merit Award system was set up with four grades: C, B, A, and A plus. The award represented a permanent increase in income. A special medical committee was set up in the Ministry to gather information on consultants throughout the country who would be deserving of such an award. The A and A plus categories actually doubled the consultant's salaries, creating an official elite in British medicine. Furthermore, the deliberations of the committee and the selection of recipients for awards are not publicized: "It would cause unnecessary jealousness and invidious comparison." This arrangement is in one sense an anomaly in British government which makes a strong case for public accountability of tax money; at the same time it is not an anomaly considering the persisting elitism of British society even in an increasingly welfare state. The arrangement was justified by this philosophy from a Royal Commission on Remuneration in 1960:". . . We consider the awards system a practical and imaginative way of securing a reasonable differentiation of income and providing relatively high earnings for the "significant minority." [18]

Another continuation of British philosophy was the specifications for the composition and responsibilities of the Regional Hospital Boards, and the Hospital Management Committees below the Boards. Fourteen Boards were established (later fifteen) in England and Wales, and 387 Hospital Management Committees. The same application can be made to Local Executive Councils for general practitioners, dentists, and pharmacists, but observations of the Regional Boards will suffice. The Regional Hospital Boards were made up of unpaid volunteers: citizens and professionals decided upon jointly by the regions and the Ministry of Health. In the course of events, naturally, these citizens and professionals came from the upper social and economic classes. The Boards have paid administrative staffs.

The traditional and worthy political theory is that responsible citizens who are assumed to have the public interest at heart can be a buffer between the state and the rank-and-file citizens for whom the Service is designed. These volunteers can work in some sort of partnership with the authorities; in the case of the National Health Service, they represent, in a new setting, a continuation of the upper class *noblesse oblige* atmosphere of the governing boards of the now nationalized voluntary hospitals. Unlike the former boards, however, the Regional Hospital Boards have no financial authority, nor, of course, are the members expected to contribute money as in the old days. The seeming anomaly then emerges of a Board responsible for planning and administration but with no fiscal responsibility; the latter lies with the Treasury. In British thinking, however, this arrangement does not seem odd. Great Britain is still a country tied together by class and custom rather than the *quid pro quo* contrac-

[18] Royal Commission on Doctors' and Dentists' Remuneration (1960), p. 81.

tual relationships of the United States and Sweden.

Why did the concept of the National Health Service emerge as it did? Its comprehensiveness and its general tax revenue source of funding are peculiarly un-British according to all standard attributes of the British style of solving problems. Even though it fell short of a state medicine system—which is the end of a continuum running from pure private practice to a completely nationalized health services system, the National Health Service is still an anomaly among British ways of doing things, what somebody referred to as an "elegant muddling through." In a seemingly authoritarian and socialistic fashion, the country went the whole hog for the works all at once, a most unusual political performance, the euphoria of World War II notwithstanding.

But on further reflection and based on a few clues from British historians and social observers, the National Health Service seems logical in the British context after all, although the administrative style continues to be what is regarded as typically British—a minimum of technical data and pride in best judgments by people who are not technical experts but are "experienced" and "well-rounded." This logic flows from two very strong influences in British history and society: aristocratic *noblesse oblige* and Christian Socialism. Both of them entertain a philosophy of help to the poor minus the grudging and puritan methods of the emerging middle class after 1832 as revealed in the Poor Laws. Aristocratic *noblesse oblige* and Christian Socialism did not think in piecemeal program terms for subsistence and medical care. In the case of medical care, the poorer classes were seen as needing comprehensiveness, not particular services or assistance for particular high-cost episodes. The underlying attitude was benevolence and paternalism, in contrast to the Liberal view of limited insurance. If the liberals had remained a dominant party instead of being split between the Conservatives and Labour after 1920, England might have continued to think in health insurance terms more or less after the American pattern, that is, by dealing with special problems rather than legislating comprehensive service all at once. Instead, England now had in the National Health Service an instrument that was meant to implement a policy of equal access to all health services by everybody. Although the existing resources would be extremely hard pressed, the concept had become "fair shares." [19]

[19] The author's interpretation is not wholly original in that various authors alluded to the underlying class and political values of distributive justice in general and he made the application to the National Health Service. Among the sources used were Lipset (1963): ". . . the noblesse oblige morality inherent in aristocracy is an aspect of collectivity-orientation. Traditionally, Britain and Australia appear to have stressed collectivity obligations more than have Can-

THE UNITED STATES

Compared to England and Sweden, the United States had an exceedingly open health services structure after World War II. By 1952, there was, in effect, a de facto decision, following the report of the President's Commission for the Health Needs of the Nation, to hold back imminent federal legislation for universal and compulsory health insurance. Thus the private sector as represented by voluntary health insurance, both the nonprofit Blue Cross and Blue Shield Plans and the for-profit insurance companies, was given an open season to see what it could do to enroll the population. It seemed that by 1952 with an administration, and a public

ada and the United States. Consequently, the rise of socialist and welfare-state concepts has placed less strain on British and Australian values than on American." (p. 280); Rose, (1964): "The testimony of one MP was 'I regard democratic Socialism as the political expression of Christianity!" (p. 23). "The rise of the Labour movement, based upon the belief in collective action for individuals ends, through trade unions, co-operatives, and the Labour Party, did not generate a conflict between individualist and collective outlook, but only between contrasting conceptions of collectivism" (p. 44). Young (1958): "The great, though temporary, contribution of socialism was that it picked out one element in the Christian teaching and gave it prominence to the exclusion of all else. It emphasized equality" (p. 128–9). De Schweinitz (1943): "In no other country has Christianity become converted to Socialism to such an extent as in Britain. In no other Socialist movement has Christian thought had such a powerful leavening influence" (p. 173). Cole and Postgate (1961): "During the 19th Century there was always a small percentage of clergymen with genuine sympathy with Socialism and the misery of the working class, whose influence prevented the church and chapels being counted wholly as enemies. Similarly, a strain of religiosity and pietism ran powerful in the Labour movement and was later to be an effective obstacle to the spread of Marxian philosophy" (p. 323). McKenzie and Silver (1968): "In the formative period of Conservative thought many Conservatives were markedly out of sympathy with the ethos of the new industrial capitalism. They were therefore more disposed than were the Liberals to champion factory legislation, limitations on hours of work, and the legal recognition of trade unions. Since these employers lacked the benevolent paternalism of the hereditary landlord, then the paternalistic state must intervene to protect the legitimate rights of the working class" (p. 30). Finally, more or less underpinning all the observations in the foregoing quotations and preceding them by 60 years or so, Dicey (reprinted 1963) wrote: "Humanitarianism, then, was the parent, if socialism was the offspring, of the factory movement, and that movement from the first came under the guidance of the Tories" (p. 224).

for that matter, that was weary of 25 years of welfare-state development plus a costly war which entailed a great deal of government direction, the voluntary plans had a clear field. They were in an expanding economy and benefited from collective bargaining between labor and management which increased "fringe benefits," a good portion of which was health insurance.

Traditional governmental concern continued with special problems: the poor, special diseases, and special groups such as mothers and children, not to mention, of course, mental illness and tuberculosis. Furthermore, the Hospital Survey and Construction Act (Hill-Burton) was a huge and noncontroversial success as a means of stimulating more money for capital funds for hospital construction and distribution. In addition, vast sums were appropriated for medical research. The Social Security Act was the main vehicle for continued skirmishes on the part of those who wished to enlarge the scope of government in the personal health services aside from capital funding and subsidies for training grants for health personnel.[20]

From the early fifties to 1965 there was political concern with health services for two main groups in the American population: the poor and the aged. Governmental concern for the poor, as a class, had been granted in principle, although there continued to be redefinitions of who the poor were, and what should be the scope of services and methods of delivery. Health services for the poor since the inauguration of the Social Security Act in 1935 had been a matter of sharing of costs between the federal government and the states, the states being the traditional initiating and administrative units. It was not until 1957, however, that the public assistance regulations of the Social Security Act were revised so that the states could obtain matching funds to pay the providers of service as a separate budgetary item from the usual subsistence items of food, clothing, and health services. Thus was set up a separate federal-state program for health services for the poor. Before this, the states had had to do it alone.

In 1960 there was finally sufficient recognition in Congress of the existence of an undefined but real class of the population above the statutory poor. This group was able to be self-sustaining as to the predictable needs of food, clothing, and shelter and was employed, but it was unable to weather the occasional costs of health services, particularly costly epi-

[20] The exception here was medical students. The A.M.A. opposed such measures because it feared federal intrusion in medical education. Until the early 1960s the A.M.A. did not subscribe to the prevailing view that there was a physician shortage.

sodes such as surgery and other in-hospital treatment. This group was quite arbitrarily called the medically indigent, and it was reasoned that providing governmental assistance to it would help to forestall its falling into the statutory indigent class. Conceptually, of course, medical indigence can happen to a family in even the highest economic groups, provided the illness episode is sufficiently prolonged.

Some form of governmental health insurance for the aged, however, was quite a different issue. Up to around 1960, public policy in the United States had always made a clear distinction between the poor and the nonpoor for special consideration. The means test concept was pervasive. Exceptions were special population groups, such as mothers and infants or veterans, to whom the nation felt it owed a special debt. Even for veterans, there was a means test for nonservice-connected disabilities. Government had traditionally also been interested in special problems that are assumed to be dangerous to society as a whole; hence it financed communicable disease control, a sanitary environment, mental hospitals for those who by definition cannot function in society, and tuberculosis hospitals to contain the spread of an infectious disease.

Health services for the aged was an ambiguous issue in the American political context because by definition two thirds of the aged fell into the poverty class while the remainder were, again by definition, able to finance a reasonable standard of living, although the spector of the increasing probability of high-cost illness episodes would jeopardize the solvency of this group as well. Another ambiguity was that the enrollment of the aged in the expanding voluntary health insurance was appreciably lower than for the general population largely because of their severance from the labor market upon retirement. While three quarters of the population was enrolled in hospital and in-hospital physician insurance plans in the early 1960s, only about half of those 65 and over were so enrolled; and the proportion decreased rapidly with increasing age. Attempts on the part of voluntary insurance to facilitate so-called conversions of the insurance policies for retiring persons were not notably successful. Efforts were made to meet increased premiums from pooled funds put aside for the purpose and/or increased payments from the retired persons themselves. However, these efforts were a burden on prevailing voluntary health insurance funding, not to mention the aged. The increasing number and proportion of retired persons in the country who would survive 10 to 15 years, on an average, was a considerable drain on voluntary health insurance funding and required the maintenance of a high premium for health insurance policies.

Other groups began to take interest in the needs of the aged. Organized labor began to espouse government health insurance for the aged for several reasons, among them to remove this expensive group from collective bargaining for health service fringe benefits. Management began to shift views for basically the same motive. Middle-class and middle-aged America was beginning to educate its children at the same time that it was becoming increasingly responsible for aged parents. It seems reasonable to generalize that because of all these conditions the middle classes began to support some sort of government health insurance for the aged, to take them off their individual backs and make them a collective responsibility.

The several years before the passage of the Medicare Act in 1965 shifted swiftly from a debate over the principle to a debate over the implementation of the principle—scope of service, sources and amounts of funding, methods of administering payments and so on. While Democrats in Congress normally were in the lead for health insurance for the aged, in due course Republicans scrambled on the bandwagon; during the final session of Congress political lines had homogenized into a rather impressive consensus, and the only remaining interest group maintaining its opposition to the last was the American Medical Association which clung to the concept of a means test. The A.M.A. was simply overwhelmed, however, particularly when it offered as a countermeasure a physician's service plan financed by the federal and state governments for the aged below a certain income. While it had appeared that the Medicare bill would be primarily a hospital and related institution measure, this counterproposal by the A.M.A. pulled the physician into the legislation when the House Appropriations Committee suggested that insurance for physicians' services be voluntary and hospital insurance compulsory. Through compulsory social security deductions the government financed institutional care. Through general revenue the government financed one half of the premium for physicians' services for the aged who elected this insurance, and paid the other half themselves. As it turned out, about 98 percent of the aged on Medicare opted for coverage of physicians' services.[21]

With the enactment of Medicare, the framework of public policy

[21] In addition to the *Uneasy Equilibrium* (Anderson, 1968), there are three other publications that can be consulted for similar details and generalizations. One is Sundquist (1968), especially Chapter VII, "For the Old, Health Care," pp. 282–321. The other are Skidmore (1970) and Chapter I, "Medicare and the Evolution of a Law," in Somers and Somers (1967), pp. 1–24. In reviewing other public issues, Sundquist shows that fundamental shifts in public policy consensus providing a framework for specific legislation occur in cycles of a generation as a result of new politicians, and new obligations, around new issues regarded as fundamental.

shifted from one of government concern with those only below a certain income to a policy breakthrough where a portion of the population came under a compulsory health insurance program, regardless of means, simply because it was above a certain age. The Medicare Act became the cutting edge of public policy regarding compulsory health insurance for the entire population simply by juggling the age groups that might come under the umbrella of the Social Security Act.

It was to be expected, given the structure of hospital and physicians' services in the United States, that the government had to turn to the private sector and negotiate and buy services from it. This was done through Blue Cross and Blue Shield Plans and selected private insurance companies acting as the administrative agents for the hospitals and physicians according to ground rules worked out between them and the social security administration, the primary administrative agency of the federal government. Thus Medicare was mainly a payment mechanism for the prevailing structure of practice. There was hardly any alternative to serve almost 20 million aged quickly. Needless to say, Medicare has already been costly beyond predictions, which were naive to begin with—a familiar pattern everywhere.

SWEDEN

After universal and compulsory health insurance legislation was put into effect in 1955 for physicians' services and drugs outside the hospital, Sweden had a rather well-defined framework in which to continue to absorb and work out the ever-accelerating pressures on the health services structure. The chief structural step was a plan to regionalize the hospital system into seven regions but with counties and municipalities retaining control and ownership and the state entering into assistance for selected elaborate facilities that the base hospitals would need. Since the base hospitals were already associated with medical schools and since these schools are owned by the state, this structural shift was smooth.

This relatively brief description of the situation in Sweden should suffice until the generic problems for all three systems are discussed. Great Britain established its public policy in 1946 in its National Health Service and thus she has had a rather clear-cut framework in which to carry out the mandate from that day on. Sweden established its framework in 1955 and the United States in 1965 when the Medicare Act was passed. It can be seen that the countries have been arranged not only chronologically but also in relation to the openness and fluidity of continuing changes: Great Britain, being the most structured, has the fewest options.[22] Sweden is certainly a more open system than is Great Britain though less so than the United States. The latter is just beginning to be pushed into more structuring by the Medicare Act, regional planning legislation, and other measures. There can, of course, never be a finished system, given the continuing development of medical knowledge and technology. However, one system can appear to be more finished than another at any given point in time.

[22] No value judgment is intended that an open system is in and of itself inherently desirable.

PART THREE

ORGANIZATION AND PERFORMANCE
FROM 1950 TO 1970 [1]

THIS PART ATTEMPTS TO DELINEATE the major characteristics of the health services in the three countries including facilities, personnel, and sources of funds. The performance of the three systems will be revealed by the trends in the use of services, expenditures, and the "payoff" for society according to some selected criteria. This will be done in the time frame of 1950–1970, or as close to 1970 as the most recent availability of data permits.

The year 1950 was selected as the starting date because by this time all three health systems had absorbed the main developments in medical knowledge and technology following World War II. It is felt, with confidence, that the sources for statistical information—both official and private—have been exhaustive. The data presented in the text, however, are selective in keeping with the general framework that has been developed. Rather than calculate detailed expenditure data breakdowns annually since 1950, it was judged in most instances that every five years would be sufficient to show gross trends and differences between the

---

[1] The statistical data throughout this book have been gathered and organized by my associate, Joanna Kravits. Since much interpolation was necessary to obtain accurate comparisons, extensive explanations and references have been provided in the Appendix tables.

three countries. Those who wish more detail will need to go to the same sources. Undoubtedly, there are those who would like to see trend data right up to 1972. Unfortunately, Swedish and British official statistical data are not published until two or more years after the event. In any case, this book is not intended to be an up-to-date source book on health service statistics in the three countries but rather a conceptual framework in which trend data are analyzed. The very currency of data is then not important unless there have been tremendous shifts in trends during the last year or so. This has not been the case.

The chapters that follow describe in detail each of the countries within a rather broad model. Model building at this stage has to be so broad that direct cause and effect as to reasons for the differences and similarities in organization and performance cannot be shown. It is hoped, however, that a framework can be presented in which further investigation can take place as more data become available. Comparisons between different systems will help to establish points of reference outside of each particular system. So far, with few exceptions, each system has been its own reference point.

A health service system can be conceptualized as shown in the figure. It has two main components:

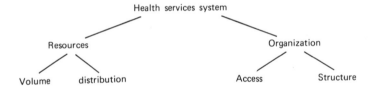

Resources. The resources of the system are the labor and capital allocated to health services in each country. These would include health personnel, structures in which health care are provided, and equipment and materials used. Resources can be viewed as having two components of importance to the understanding of how people use health services: (1) total volume of resources available relative to population and (2) geographical distribution of these resources. Resources are presented as national aggregates with some attention to distribution.

Organization. This term simply describes what the system does with its resources. It deals with the manner in which personnel and facilities are coordinated and controlled in the delivery of health services. Like resources, organization can also be regarded as consisting chiefly of two components: access and structure. Access refers to the means by which the patient gains entry to the health services system and the pathways of the treatment process within it. It specifies the criteria that must be met before medical care at varying levels is received. The degree of access in any system varies according to such things as charges for services that must be paid directly by the patient and length of the queue for various kinds of treatment.

Structure, the second component of organization, deals with characteristics of the system which determine what happens to the patient once entry to the system is gained. Among the elements under structure would be the practice habits of primary practitioners who see the patient first, the utilization of auxiliary services, the process of referrals to other sources of care, and admission criteria to hospitals.

At this stage of knowledge of the organization and performance of the health services, it is very clear that the structural component is the most difficult of the health services to define and to relate to utilization patterns and impact on health indices. The structural component is highly interrelated with other components. Access in turn depends in part on structure, and the structure of any system is dependent on the resources made available.

An extremely important overall assumption is that the greater the understanding we have of the structural component—what happens inside of the system once a patient gains entry—the better basis we have for making comparisons between systems as well as for describing single systems. A fascinating datum is that the proportion of the population who see a physician at least once during a year in the United States, Sweden, and England, is the same: two thirds. Use patterns after a patient sees a physician in the three countries vary considerably indicating a host of factors that affect the use of services differentially in each country. Reasons for such differences are by no means clear. Some are undoubtedly structural while others relate to the social characteristics of each country.

VII

Organizational Characteristics of
Facilities, Personnel, and
Funding

It may not seem valid at first glance to compare three countries that vary so much in population and land space: the United States with a population of over 200 million and a land area of over 3 million square miles; Sweden with a population of 8 million and 174,000 square miles; and England (and Wales) with nearly 50 million people in a land area of 58,000 square miles. Furthermore, the rates of population growth have been unequal. The fastest growing country since 1950 has been the United States, where the population has increased by a third in less than 20 years while Sweden and England and Wales experienced only a 10 percent increase each. These growth data are important because of the strains that such growth places on the absorptive capacity of the health systems in the three countries.

The United States has had the largest population growth and has by far the largest land area. It also reveals the greatest extremes in population densities from 26,000 people per square mile in New York City to three per square mile in Wyoming. Stockholm and London metropolitan areas have less than half the density of New York City, while the northernmost county of Sweden, with eight people per square mile, is more dense than Wyoming. England has a relatively high density everywhere.

Still, it is of significance as a common basis for comparing health systems that the three countries are quite close together in proportions of the population living in urban areas: United States 70 percent; Sweden 77; and England and Wales 80. It is this common level of economic development that lends validity to comparisons, as this level is reflected in levels of living, gross national product, and social surpluses available for a wide variety of social needs. Aiding the comparisons is the fact that general health conditions as revealed by the standard health indices fall into similar patterns of leading causes of death and similar broad patterns of prevailing morbidity.

It is not so much the size of the population or the land area that is crucial in international comparisons as the feasibility of showing that there are definable social systems and social organizational characteristics prevailing in any country. Health services organizations reveal an essentially typical pattern from area to area, peculiar to each country. In the United States, for example, the autonomous voluntary hospital and the autonomous and privately practicing physician plus certain public measures for the poor and various forms of health insurance for the self-sustaining elements of the population are the pattern all over the country with variations only in degree and proportions. The pattern in Sweden is county- and municipality-owned hospitals, free to patients and with salaried physicians, and private physicians practicing outside of the hospitals and paid fees by the government insurance funds. In England the uniform pattern is the hospital owned and funded by the central government with salaried physicians on its staff and general practitioners outside of the hospital paid by capitation by the central government. Now for more details to fill in the broad strokes in the foregoing description.

ENGLAND

The main organizational and structural features of the British system can be summed up as follows. The National Health Service has three parallel divisions reporting to the Minister of Health and Social Security who in turn is a member of the cabinet, and a member of the House of Commons of the party in power. Fiscally, the Treasury wields tremendous power in the allocation of funds to the numerous enterprises in which modern governments are engaged. The first of the three parallel divisions consists of the hospitals which include the specialists in a salaried hierarchy topped by a consultant for each specialty who is allotted a certain number of beds under his control. The hospitals are divided into 15 regions (in England and Wales) with a population base ranging from two million to five million people. Each region has at least one teaching hospital as a referral facility for serious, relatively infrequent, and complicated cases. The teaching hospitals are not part of the regional hospital governing body but are a separate fiscal and administrative entity reporting directly to the Minister. In each hospital region the top governing body is the Regional Hospital Board. The members of the Board are appointed through joint consultations with the Minister and the parties at interest in the region and represent the usual range of constituencies: medical, dental, pharmaceutical, and prominent citizens. They serve without pay and carry enormous responsibilities in that they are to review the distribution, delivery, and costs of hospital based services, including regional blood banks, for example, and the maintenance, improvement, and construction of hospital facilities. An annual budget to this end is submitted to the Minister. The Regional Hospital Board has no taxing power and very few methods of raising funds for operating or capital purposes outside of the general tax revenues carefully watched by the Treasury. Hence it is in the anomalous position of having responsibility to deliver a service without the power to relate finance to delivery. Within the overall regional budget the Board may juggle the number and kind of personnel, but it has no control over salary ranges. These are established nationally and with a few exceptions are uniform throughout England and Wales. The Board hires all medical personnel and has a paid and permanent administrative staff headed by an executive officer and, parallel to the executive officer, a fiscal officer, both of whom report to the Board. There is no stipulation as to whether the executive officer be a physician or a nonmedical administrator. In the paid administrative hierarchy the top jobs in the Regional Hospital Board are regarded highly in the health administrative career ladder. The incumbents handle hundreds of millions of dollars and affect the hospital services for an average of three million people.

Under the Regional Hospital Board there are a number of hospital units called Hospital Management Committees which are concerned with the daily operation of hospitals within their jurisdictions. The Management Committees report to the Regional Hospital Board. Again, as with the Regional Hospital Boards, the Management Committees are made up of unpaid members appointed in joint consultation with the local groups at interest and the Regional Hospital Board. The interests represented are medical, dental, pharmaceutical, and other professional and business groups. The Management Committee has a paid and permanent staff headed by an executive officer. This administrative staff works rather intensively with the various hospitals and departments within hospitals in its jurisdictions. Each hospital has exceedingly little autonomy in staffing, facilities, and equipment. These are controlled by the Hospital Management Committees who in turn report to the Regional Hospital Board, the fundamental and pervasive control being, of course, fiscal.

There is general agreement that this hospital organizational structure has enormously improved the distribution of specialists. There is also some agreement that, even though few hospitals have been built since 1946, there has been an upgrading of hospitals so that the minimum standard is now higher than it might have been without a regionalized hospital system, although the very top quality may have been inhibited. In other words the range in quality has been narrowed by upgrading. The foregoing shifts have been made possible by central control over finances, and then, within each regional hospital board, control over allocations within the region. There has been no master plan as conceived by theories of planners but rather a filling out of gross and obvious gaps in the hospital system that the National Health Service took over in 1946.

The British like the Americans (and the Swedes) plan rather gently even though the Minister has enormous power both theoretically and legally. The political traditions in the three countries are so similar that arbitrary directives are unacceptable; hence there is a great amount of consultation between the parties at interest before a policy basic to the functioning of the hospital system is applied. If in England the Minister began to issue directives in the style of the system in the U.S.S.R., the whole informal structure of understandings and agreements on which the formal structure depends would collapse. This is not to say that in the long haul the British social and political system might not evolve to that type of arbitrariness, but it is far from this situation now.[1] The chief control, broadside as it may be, but pervasive and visible enough for all to see and accommodate to quite gracefully, is the amount of money ultimately allowed by the Treasury. Given this fact, the lightening rod for dissatisfaction with the amount of money for facilities, equipment, personnel, and salaries is the Treasury, backed up, of course, by Parliament. Seen by an American, it presents a tight administrative and fiscal operation, but then the United States has other problems.

The second administratively and fiscally parallel division is the Local Executive Councils, 134 of them in England and Wales, with population bases ranging from 15,000 to over three million. These administrative and fiscal units are concerned with the general practitioner and dental and pharmaceutical services. It is this unit that contracts with the foregoing providers and pays them. As with the hospital service, each Local Ex-

---

[1] See, for example, an excellent study of the legal implications of the National Health Service: Southwick (1968).

ecutive Council has an appointed membership which is unpaid. Such membership has a heavy emphasis on the health professionals plus the usual members of business, labor, the church, and upper-class segments of British society. There is a paid and permanent administrative staff. The patient lists of the general practitioner panels are maintained by this administrative unit, since the practitioner is paid at an annual rate per capita for each person who has selected him. The panel limit is 3500 patients per physician. The capitation fee is the main source of income for general practitioners, but additional sources are mileage, fees for maternity services and immunizations, and practice allowances for premises. There is some allowance made for the age composition of a panel. The Local Executive Council maintains grievance machinery, particularly regarding general practitioner services for patients.

In addition to general practitioners, the Councils have jurisdiction over dentists and pharmacists. The dentists are paid for each service according to a negotiable fee schedule plus a charge paid by the patient at the beginning of a service period. The pharmacists are paid for each prescription (plus a charge paid by the patient) according to a negotiated price schedule.

The third parallel division in the National Health Service is the Local Health Councils. These are actually the original local public health agencies which depended for financing mainly on local tax rates the traditional public health functions of which were made part of the National Health Service structure. The Local Health authorities are headed by public health officers who are physicians and normally trained in public health as well. The governing body for the Local Health Councils is the locally elected county councillors. This, then, is the only division of the three in the National Health Service that has an elected governing body.

These departments are charged with sanitary environmental control, communicable disease control, and maternal and child health services. The assumption is that the local public health departments are to work in cooperation with the local general practitioners, who are to avail themselves of the public health nurses and home visitors for their patients. The initiative for those services is to come from the practitioners. Maternal and child health clinics are at the initiative of the local health departments with no particular reference to the local general practitioners on whose panels the mothers and children are enrolled. One-half of the funding for public health services is from local property taxation; the other half is a subsidy from the Ministry of Health.

The Local Health Council Jurisdictions have no necessary relationship to the jurisdictions of the Local Executive Councils responsible for the general practitioners, dental, and pharmaceutical services. Nor is there any necessary jurisdictional relationship of the Local Executive Councils to the Regional Hospital Board. Since these three parallel divisions have their own budgets and their own boards reporting directly to the Minister, there is no administrative necessity for exactly similar jurisdictions as far as the Ministry is concerned.

The reasons for the creation of the tripartite structure have been presented previously, but continuation of these divisions has been a source of endless discussion since the National Health Service was established.[2] The creation of the Service itself was, of course, regarded as a fundamental step toward the rationalization of the apparent confusion it was to correct and the facilitation of overall planning, coordination, and integration of the total services. The three parallel divisions have been regarded as a major obstacle to the ultimate coordination and integration of the health services from home visitors to the dazzling medical technology of the major teaching hospitals.

The logical system would consist of one regional district for all personal and public health services, under one governing board, with one budget, and with one administrative officer and staff so that "national" allocations of personnel, facilities, and money could be made under central direction, with each such district reporting to the Minister. Indeed, this is now in the form of a White Paper.[3]

Finally, as to the exceedingly important question of amount and sources of funding, approximately 85 percent of the total budget comes from general tax revenue, most of which in turn comes from the personal

---

[2] The case of the pregnant woman who falls between the allegedly wide cracks of the tripartite structure is now part of the stock of case stories that emerged during the development and operation of the health services system. She will determine pregnancy by going to her general practitioner on whose panel she is listed (Local Executive Council); a conscientious practitioner will refer her to the local public health nurse for periodic visits during pregnancy (Local Health Councils). During the pregnancy period she experiences complications and her practitioner refers her to a specialist (Regional Hospital Board). Upon discharge by the specialist she returns presumably to the public health nurse and the general practitioner. When her labor pains start, she might be delivered at home (Local Executive Council) or in a hospital (Regional Hospital Board). Incidentally, 80 percent of the births are now delivered in the hospital. Upon discharge she returns to the general practitioner and should resume contact with the public health nurse. Should she experience postmaternity complications requiring a specialist or should the infant become ill, the "appropriate" divisions are then referred to.

[3] A government report for discussion purposes *with* a commitment to a given policy. This was preceded by two Green Papers, a government report for discussion purposes *without* commitment to a given policy.

income tax. The other 15 percent of the budget derives from a variety of sources.

SWEDEN

The Swedish health services have been informally regionalized for a long time because of county and major municipality responsibility for the ownership, funding, and operation of the hospitals. The counties and cities with university hospitals served as referral centers.

It is only since World War II that the counties and municipalities have been faced with the tremendous investment and manpower requirements of an expanding medical technology beyond their capacity. In a sense, Sweden also has a tripartite structure of public health officers, out-of-hospital practitioners, and the hospitals. Until recently the public health officers were state functionaries who also practiced medicine. Since 1961 they have become part of the county and major municipality health services, that is, the hospitals and the public health officers. The health officers are in charge of the usual public health activities of sanitary environmental control, communicable disease control, maternal and infant welfare, and public health nurses and nurse-midwives. The physicians outside of the hospital and public health departments, comprising almost one third of the physicians in Sweden, are autonomous entrepreneurs. Since 1955 the income for private practitioners comes essentially from the compulsory health insurance act relating to out-of-hospital (including hospital outpatient departments) physicians' services.

The health insurance act is administered by an insurance department in the central government through about 600 sickness-insurance funds which pay the physicians and pharmacists. The central government collects payroll deductions from employers and employees, contributes a portion itself, and distributes this money to the sickness-insurance funds in accordance with the number of physicians, would-be patient population, and past experience. These funds are responsible for their own solvency.

The physicians have no contractural arrangement with the sickness-insurance funds. It is understood, but not necessarily adhered to by the physicians, that they are paid around three fourths of a fee schedule set by the fund with the patient paying the remainder. For specialists in private practice and outside of the hospital, the patient is reimbursed for approximately one half of a higher fee norm set by the fund. Thus the financial relationship between the physician and patient remains that of private practice, and the patient sends his claim for the costs of services to the nearest sickness-insurance fund. The public health officer is in the same fiduciary relationship, the exception being that he has to abide by a set free schedule. (In January, 1970, health officers were put on full salary; this is explained in Chapter XII.)

Drugs and medicines are provided by the government contracting with the retail pharmacies at negotiated prices. Normally, the patient pays one half of the charge for prescriptions for all except lifesaving drugs which are free of charge. Standards and prices are regulated.

In comparison with the British system, the Swedish health system is quite decentralized as to variety of sources of funding, ownership of facilities, and the relative autonomy of the primary practitioners outside of the hospital. The patient has a wide range of options as to where to enter the system: a general practitioner, a specialist on the staff of the hospital or one whose practice is outside of the hospital, a hospital outpatient department or polyclinic affording no choice of physician but at least a guaranteed limit on the fee, or a public health officer in areas outside of the cities.

Funding for the hospitals and associated medical and other supporting staff and the public health portion of the health officers functions comes from the counties and major municipalities. Centrally collected funds from payroll deductions for employers and employees plus some addition by the central government pays for out-of-hospital physicians' services, diagnostic and treatment services by the public health officers, and out-of-hospital services by the hospital based specialists. These funds also pay for drugs.

The central government contributes relatively little to either capital funding or the daily operations of the county-and municipally owned hospitals. The leverage the central government has, however, on the hospitals is in its allocation of medical staff throughout the country. The National Medical Board determines staffing ratios and quality criteria. Hence, while a county can actually build or expand a hospital, it better not do so unless it is assured of medical staff by the National Board. Portentous as this form of control may appear to local autonomy, the issue has so far never arisen.

There would certainly be general agreement that the Swedish hospitals are of a rather uniform and high minimum quality regardless of geographic area. Perhaps the local pride of counties and municipalities can account for this uniformity. Fundamentally, it would seem to be a reflection of the general Swedish culture in which the hospitals did not emerge from a class system like England's or from a more or less market concept as in the United States. The momentum for excellence in Sweden has continued in the face of enormously rising costs. It remains to be seen what the breakoff point may be as social priorities are reappraised.

THE UNITED STATES

Compared with England and Sweden, the health services structure of the United States appear chaotic, or can be described as a visiting English economist described American society in general: "riotous pluralism." [4] Still, as we go further into studies of the structural and dynamic characteristics of the American health services, there is more structure than appears on the surface because of the sheer necessity for some sort of informal regularity of patterns of use, referrals, financing, and programming.

The English and Swedish systems are not functionally as tidy as they appear in their easily described formal structures. As one delves more deeply into the processes of the two systems and shucks off the formal structures, the medical technological developments common to all three countries reveal quite similar processes irrespective of the formal structures. Research on the use of, expenditures for, and organization of the American health services has been far more extensive than that for England and Sweden, or any other country for that matter. Such studies have revealed distinct and repetitive patterns through time and areas.[5]

The backbone of the American health services system is the voluntary hospital and the privately practicing physician who in most instances has admission privileges to a hospital. The hospitals and physicians continue to be autonomous in their capital funding and their daily operations as to charges and fees. The trend is toward some constriction of this freedom by the large buyers of services, particularly the federal government for Medicare patients, who now pay approximately 30 percent of total expenditures for health services. Hospital medical association-sponsored Blue Cross and Blue Shield Plans and private insurance companies pay for approximately 80 percent of the voluntary hospital charges and 40 percent of the physicians' charges, mainly those for surgery. Capital funding for hospitals comes from federal matching funds which stimulate the

---

[4] Shonfield (1969), p. 323.

[5] Andersen and Anderson (1967), Andersen, Smedby, and Anderson (1970), Anderson, Collette, and Feldman (1963), Anderson and Feldman (1956), Anderson and Kravits (1968), Anderson and Sheatsley (1959, 1967), Falk et al. (1933), McNerney (1962).

creation of private fund drives, now beginning to be supplemented by borrowing.

The range of options by which patients can enter the system is wide, the main entry points being the general practitioner, the internist, the pediatrician, the eye-ear-nose and throat specialist, and the obstetrician-gynecologist. Despite easy access to specialists, 41 percent of the adult population still report a general practitioner as their regular physician.[6]

Both hospitals and physicians have incomes from a variety of sources, avoiding a single source of funds. This system is an integral outgrowth of the private and nonprofit sector of the American economy. The public health programs described for England and Sweden are hardly as widespread and systematically offered to the entire population in the United States. Public health has a distinctly lower-income clientele for all but its sanitary environmental activities. For the great majority of the population, immunization and maternal and infant care are carried out by the private practitioners.

It should not be inferred from the foregoing description that the American health services system is static and that it will remain more or less this way for the indefinite future. Its very looseness and diversity promises a great deal of change structurally and financially on the local level, but the direction of this change is difficult to direct because of the diffusion of ownership and sources of funds. The government owns nothing, so to speak; hence it has to buy services from the voluntary health structure once it is given a mandate as in Medicare. Thus it is in a position to use its power of the purse to induce changes in the system. In England, in contrast, the government owns the facilities and is a monopoly employer of the physicians and other health personnel. In Sweden there is more diffusion: local governments own the hospitals, hire associated personnel, and can move the hospital system into some kind of coordinated and regional relationship in their bargaining relationship with the central government.

TREND DATA

This section presents trends in facilities, personnel, and sources of funds in the three countries from 1950 to as close to 1970 as sources permit. Subsequent chapters provide trend data on use and expenditures.

---

[6] Andersen and Anderson (1967), p. 13.

Funding, Facilities, and Personnel

The extent to which funding is decentralized or centralized is of extreme importance in the financing of health services. What may be the happy balance is, of course, open to continuous debate. It can be concluded that more money is better than less money for the health services, because no one knows how to define "adequate." It should be made clear, however, that this judgment is made about expenditures for personal health services and not for traditional public health services such as sanitary environment and communicable disease control. Expenditures for the latter can be quite reasonably estimated in relation to investment and outcome. There is evidence that a diversity of sources of funds does add up to a larger total than if there is a dominant or single source of funds which has to be directly and visibly competitive with other national priorities.[7] This assumption is naturally limited to countries that are relatively affluent and have some leeway, private or public, for social priorities.

In ascending order of centralization of funding—the United States, Sweden, and England—the gross trends in the degree of centralization of sources of funding and the proportioning among various sources of funding are seen in Table 2 for the period from 1950 to 1965 or later. In the main, the division between private and public sectors is self-evident. The private sector comprises funds that came from patients paying for services directly or from voluntary private health insurance paying on their behalf. The public sector implies that there is an element of compulsion in the collecting of funds through whatever means: payroll deductions, sales taxes, or personal income taxes. In any case, whatever their sources in the private or public sectors in the three countries under study, these funds must come from the essentially privately owned economy producing the social surpluses necessary to finance a variety of health and welfare measures. The respective governments are keenly aware of this and in essence leave the revenue producing private enterprises alone to pursue their profit-oriented ends as long as a politically negotiated part of the profit or surplus can be collected to serve public ends as defined by politically mandated health and welfare programs.

In a state-owned economic system such as that in the U.S.S.R., it is the state authorities who determine what surpluses will be allocated to certain ends, and the private and public sectors do not exist. Western Liber-

---

[7] In addition to the evidence in this book see also Abel-Smith (1967).

TABLE 2 PERCENT DISTRIBUTION OF SOURCES OF FUNDS
FOR HEALTH CARE EXPENDITURES

Country and Year	Private				Public			Grand Total
	Patient	Insurance	Other	Total	Central	Local	Total	
United States (1950)	57	9	6	72	13	15	28	100
Sweden (1950)	16	6	—	22	26	52	78	100
England (1950)	15	—	—	15	79	6	85	100
United States (1969)	35	19	8	62	25	13	38	100
Sweden (1965)	15	—	—	15	31	54	85	100
England (1965)	15	a	—	15	80	5	85	100

Source: Tables A2 and A3.
a Less than one half of 1 percent.

116

al-Democratic countries, however, are in a constant political debate about the appropriate working relationships between the private and public sectors. The health services in the United States, Sweden, and England clearly reflect this debate historically and currently, as Table 2 illustrates.

The table also shows an overall dichotomy in the sources of funds between the private and the public sectors. More than one third of the funding for health services in the United States now comes from the various levels of government. In both Sweden and England only 15 percent of total funding is *not* from government mandate. Between 1950 and the latter part of the 1960s the United States shifted from 28 percent public to 38 percent public funding chiefly because of the enactment of Medicare and some increased expenditures for the poor through Medicaid which was enacted at the same time. Prior to 1965 the proportions of funds from private and public sources had remained stable since the thirties—75 percent private and 25 percent public—revealing a public policy consensus as to the role of government in the health services which was eventually broken through by Medicare.

Within both the private and public sectors in the United States significant shifts in sources of funds were taking place which estalished the base for a pluralism of sources. Within the private sector in 1950, four fifths of the funds came from patients directly at time of service, and only 13 percent from voluntary health insurance. Within the public sector slightly less than half of the funds were from the federal government and slightly more than half from the states and counties, mainly the states. Within the private sector, by 1969, only 56 percent of the funds came from patients directly and a third from rapidly growing voluntary health insurance. Within the public sector, the federal government was contributing almost twice as much as state and local governments.

In 1950 expenditures from the public sector were for traditional public responsibilities for the health services of the people: public health departments, mental hospitals and tuberculosis hospitals, public medical care for the poor, war veterans, and a capital subsidy for the construction and renovation of hospitals. The enactment of Medicare in 1965 represented a distinct public policy breakthrough in that a group of people were covered regardless of income level.

It can be seen that the providers of services in the United States have a variety of sources of income which they can integrate into their operations in some way. The most important shift in sources of funds has, of course, been from the patient directly to a third party. Fully one half of the income of hospitals is from government, about 40 percent is from voluntary health insurance, and the remainder from patients directly. Within health insurance, about one half of payments are from Blue Cross and the other half from a myriad of private insurance companies. It is estimated that close to three quarters of the cost of group health insurance is contributed by employers as a fringe benefit. This fringe benefit evolved largely from the normal collective bargaining process. The tax-exempt status of payroll deductions encourages both labor and management to enlarge the fringe benefits. Now, however, both labor and management are becoming restive regarding the rising costs of health services and the necessity for increasing payroll deductions.

The foregoing analysis can be repeated for physicians although they do not experience the same proportioning of sources of funds. This depends in part on the specialty. Hospital-related specialists such as surgeons receive a major portion of their incomes from third parties, perhaps as high as three quarters, but within this percentage the major portion comes from voluntary health insurance. The physicians have their own medical society-sponsored Blue Shield plans which possibly provide one half of the income from voluntary health insurance, with the other half coming from a myriad of private insurance companies. On an average for all physicians, even those with specialties that must be hospital related, it is likely that only 10 percent of their income comes from government. An appreciable portion still comes from patients at time of service, perhaps as high as one half.

Compared with the United States, Sweden and England appear to be models of simplicity, as indeed they are, but there is still some degree of diffusion, particularly in Sweden. In the American sense, Sweden and England have eliminated the relative importance of the private sector so that it is a residual of the larger system rather than a more than equal partner as in the United States.

In 1950 the public sector in Sweden was 7 percentage points smaller than in 1965 (78 and 85 percent respectively) because in 1955 Sweden inaugurated a compulsory health insurance plan for out-of-hospital physicians' services. In 1950 voluntary health insurance for such physicians' services accounted for 6 percent of the total expenditures. Thus by 1965 the sources of funds for the Swedish health services were 15 percent from the patient directly, 31 percent from the central government, and 54 percent from the counties and municipalities. Voluntary health insurance was, therefore, eliminated and does not exist in Sweden today, not because it is forbidden but apparently because there is no market. The 15 percent from the patient is arbitrarily classified as private sector in that it represents the proportion of funds paid by the patients, but it is not private in the American sense. It is made up of small payments at time of service for out-of-hospital physicians' services (25 percent for general practitioner and 50 percent for specialist), partial payment for prescribed drugs, and full payment for uncovered services such as dental care for adults, appliances, and unprescribed drugs. Thus charges to the patient can be regarded as an administrative tool to control volume, provide leeway for physicians' incomes, and provide a source of income for the system. There is obviously hardly any power balance between the private and public sectors as in the United States.

In Sweden, however, there is a significant balance between the central government and the counties, as seen in the proportions of sources of funding. The counties and municipalities control the hospitals and employ the associated physicians; the central government does not own anything and controls indirectly through standards and medical staffing. Ostensibly, the central government could control the out-of-hospital physicians through its insurance department and the 600 or so local sickness-insurance societies. The central government is the collection agency for payroll deductions from employer and employees to which it adds a more or less equal portion from general tax revenue and distributes this fund to the local insurance societies who in turn pay the physicians and the pharmacists. The proportion of payroll deductions from the employer and employees and contributions by the central government are matters for political negotiations, because the government has to authorize the tax collection. It should be noted that on any matters involving collective bargaining the government is automatically a party at interest to preserve its fiscal integrity in relation to the overall economy. The government is not an arbitrator—a function (and power) that labor and management have been loath to give government since a famous agreement between labor and management in 1938 to forestall compulsory arbitration.

Since 1948, when the National Health Service Act went into effect, the sources of funding for the health services in England have remained almost unchanged. As has been noted, 80 percent of the health services are financed by the central government, almost all through general tax revenue but with a very small part from employer-employee deductions. Only 5 percent comes from local government and that chiefly for the public health services, a remnant of the historical responsibility of the local government for such services, which are now also subsidized by the central government. The 15 percent of the total that comes from the patient directly at time of service is partially, as in Sweden, a function of the National Health Service itself, to control services or collect revenue outside of the National Health Service. This mixture of charges on prescriptions and dental care, charges for appliances, and extra charges for so-called amenity beds in National Health Service hospitals for those who wish to pay for privacy. Most of the 15 percent, however, is payment for strictly private medical care outside of the Health Service for private consultants and private hospitals. Less than 1 percent of the funds comes from voluntary health insurance, although in 1950 there was not even this much to report. Private health insurance has been growing during the past 10 years and now covers about 5 million people, chiefly for specialist services and private accommodations. Within the British context private health insurance is an interesting phenomenon because health insurance benefits are formulated in relation to the National Health Service. The Service is naturally so dominant that exceedingly costly illness episodes such as brain surgery cannot be carried out without its facilities. Private health insurance is, thus, a residual and hardly a substitute.

Insofar as the control over funding enables control over the scope and depth of facilities, personnel, and services, the National Health Service is a clear example of centralized funding and legally centralized operation. Such centralized funding permits the allocation of national resources in relation to some kind of national plan: education, housing, roads, defense, and so on. Whether health service is given the resources it may need in relation to other national priorities can be (and is) a matter for endless debate. Whether national resources should be allocated by as centralized a means as is illustrated by the National Health Service can also be endlessly debated. It is hardly possible to discuss such questions rationally considering how deeply they are embedded in political ideologies rather than being simple questions of administration.

The distribution of the medical dollar, to use American terminology, is a useful means of revealing how much is spent for various items of health goods and services. There is a great deal of discussion of and concern with the concept of a "proper" distribution of expenditures for various types of goods and services.

After 75 years of quite unstinting support from both private and public sources which has made it the pride of many communities, the general hospital is now feared as a possible economic albatross in the spectrum of health services. It is absorbing a larger and larger portion of the medical dollar in all three countries, and the *per diem* costs are regarded with trepidation everywhere. Hence there is now discussion of the possibility of deemphasizing inpatient care and returning the service site to the home and office or at least to facilities such as health centers and nursing and convalescent homes.

As revealed in Table 3 it is, of course, not surprising that the hospital is the most expensive of all service components, but the differences between the three countries are striking. The United States devotes the lowest proportion of the medical dollar to the hospital, 34 percent, followed by England, 39 percent, and Sweden, 47 percent.[8] Sweden's proportion is truly high and reflects the spontaneous emphasis hospitals have received in the Swedish health system, with less emphasis on physicians. The United States devotes 22 percent of its medical dollar to physicians' services compared with Sweden and England which devote 14 and 13 percent respectively. The proportions spent for out-of-hospital drugs also vary widely—19 percent in England, 12 percent in the United States, and 8 percent in Sweden. In England such items as welfare food supplements, which would not be considered drugs in the other two countries, undoubtedly help to run up this total.

TABLE 3   PERCENT DISTRIBUTION OF EXPENDITURES BY COMPONENTS OF HEALTH SERVICE, 1965

	United States	Sweden	England
Hospital	34%	47%	39%
Physician	22	14	13
	56	61	52
Dentist	7	10	5
Drugs	12	8	19
Nursing home	3	6	4
Public health	2	2	1
Construction	5	8	5
Other	15	5	14
Total	100%	100%	100%

Source. Table A8.

Another method of analyzing the physician component is to show its proportion as a sum of the hospital, physician, and drug components. The physician is technically the sole decision maker in the use of all three components. As borne out in the foregoing discussion but made more dramatic here, in the United States expenditures for physicians' services account for 32 percent of the total compared with only 20 percent in Sweden and 18 percent in England.

Table 4 shows that for all types of hospital beds the United States, Sweden and England varied appreciably in both 1950 and 1968. The rank order of number of beds remains the same. The United States and

[8] These estimates exclude salaries of hospital-based physicians in England and Sweden to permit comparability.

TABLE 4   ALL HOSPITAL BEDS PER 1000 POPULATION,
1950 AND 1968

Country	1950	1968
United States	9.6	8.3
Sweden	14.1	16.3
England	10.4	9.6

Source. Table A22.

England reduced their total bed capacity somewhat whereas Sweden in-creased it even though she had a bed capacity roughly 50 percent in ex-cess of the other two countries. These data include all hospitals. Where general hospital beds are broken out, as in Table 5, the Swedish excess remains relatively high, currently about 30 percent more beds than either country. It is of interest, however, that Sweden increased her general hos-pital beds very slightly from 1950 to 1968, 5.7 to 5.9 beds per 1000 popu-lation, whereas the United States increased its supply appreciably, 3.3 to 4.0, and England appeared to have *reduced* her supply appreciably from 5.0 to 4.2 beds per 1000 population so that these two countries are now virtually equal. Sweden's supply of general hospital beds thus continues to be much greater than that in the other two countries and will be re-flected in her volume of comparative use.

The foregoing data can be explained, so far, only by *ex post facto* and frequently internally inconsistent explanations. There is no overarching and tested theory of what the various indicators of a health service mean. Subsequent data will continue to confirm this uncomfortable observation. Probably the most dramatic data relate to the number of personnel per patient day (excluding physicians) in general hospitals in the three coun-tries. One might reasonably assume that somehow institutions as appar-ently similar as general hospitals would require somewhat similar staffing

TABLE 5 GENERAL HOSPITAL BEDS PER 1000 POPULATION,
1950 AND 1968

Country	1950	1968
United States	3.3	4.0
Sweden	5.7	5.9
England	5.0	4.2

Source. Table A21.

ratios. But this is not so, as Table 6 shows. In 1950 the United States had the highest staff-patient day ratio, followed by England and Sweden. In 1967 the United States continued to have the highest staff-patient day ratio, 2.7, again followed by England and Sweden with 2.4 and 1.5 respectively. Why are the American and English ratios so much higher than Sweden's? How can the Swedish hospitals manage with a ratio 45 percent lower than the American? Interestingly all three countries increased their staffing ratios from 1950 to 1967—England by 60 percent, the United States by 50 percent, and Sweden by a mere 15 percent; nevertheless the direction was the same.

TABLE 6   PERSONNEL PER PATIENT DAY—SHORT-TERM GENERAL HOSPITALS

Country	1950	1967	Percent Increase
United States	1.8	2.7	50
Sweden	1.3	1.5	15
England	1.5	2.4	60

Source. Table A20.

As is true of hospital bed-population ratios, there are also significant variations in ratios of types of personnel to population. Indications then are that health systems in different countries such as those under study are able to function more or less tolerably with such variations. Table 7 shows that the differences in the number of physicians per 100,000 population was truly great in 1950 but had narrowed considerably by 1967. All three countries had increased their physician supply during the 17 years, but at different rates. Sweden's rapid pace of increase is planned to

TABLE 7   PHYSICIANS PER 100,000 POPULATION, 1950 AND 1967

Country	1950	1967	Percent Increase
United States	149	158	6
Sweden	69	117	70
England	99	119	17

Source. Table A15.

continue for several more years until it approximates the ratio of the United States. Evidence that this plan is working is that from 1967 to 1968 the Swedish physician supply increased from 117 to 124 per 100,-000 population. This great increase in Sweden reveals what can be done when there is a public policy that is implemented by central authorities. Still, the fact that the United States maintained a little better than constant ratio in face of a 25 percent increase in population reveals the possibility of providing more physicians if the intent is there.

The practice sites of physicians in the three countries as seen in Table 8 require some interpretation because of the differences in staffing arrangements for hospital-associated physicians in the United States on the one hand and Sweden and England on the other. When the proportion of physicians in private practice in the United States who have hospital admission privileges is added to those based in hospitals full time, the proportion of hospital-affiliated physicians approximates 90 percent of all physicians. The evidence is that about 87 percent of physicians in private

TABLE 8   DISTRIBUTION, BY PRIMARY SITE OF PRACTICE,
OF PHYSICIANS PROVIDING PATIENT CARE, 1967

Country	Hospital	Private Office
United States	24	76
Sweden	64	36
England	51	49

Source. Table A19.

practice do have some kind of hospital affiliation.[9] Thus a far larger proportion of American physicians actually have the privilege of admitting patients to hospitals than do physicians in either Sweden or Britain. If the estimated one tenth of English general practitioners who have some type of limited hospital admission privileges are added to the hospital-based physician total, the English proportion is increased to 61 percent of all physicians.[10] The fact that 64 percent of the Swedish physicians are

[9] Health Information Foundation (1958), p. 6. This datum is from 1955 and the proportion may well be higher in view of recent pressure of general practitioners to obtain hospital affiliations.

[10] Stevens (1966), p. 161. The proportion of general practitioners who have some kind of contact with the hospital is actually as high as 50 percent, according to Mechanic (1968) (2). Mechanic included general practitioners who

based full time in the hospitals is some indication of the emphasis that Sweden has, so far, placed on institutional care. In training more physicians, there is an attempt to increase the supply of physicians who do not have hospital appointments by keeping the number of hospital positions constant.

It is apparent that the control of the medical profession by the hospitals is diffused in the United States and rather structured in Sweden and England. The American medical profession has more autonomy individually in relation to the hospital medical staffing structure. This is not to imply that the Swedish and British hospital-based medical staffs do not exercise a great deal of power in the hospital system; they do so in a more structured and hierarchial manner than in the United States. In the United States the professional relationships of physicians with hospital affiliations is essentially collegial and equal. The professional relationships of physicians in hospitals in Sweden and England are in large part hierarchial; the collegial relationships exist mainly among the top echelon of consultants.

Table 9 gives the distribution of physicians by type of primary activity. The proportion of physicians in general practice in England, 48 percent, reflects, of course, the British attempt to maintain general practice in its pure form as the primary source of medical care for the individual and

TABLE 9   DISTRIBUTION OF PHYSICIANS BY TYPE OF
PRIMARY ACTIVITY, 1967

	United States		Sweden		England	
Patient care						
General practice	23%		35%		48%	
Specialties	70%		56%		50%	
Medical		21		26		14
Surgical		27		17		20
Other		22		13		16
Administration		7		9		2
		100%		100%		100%

Source. Table A18.

are clinical assistants to the consultants with no prerogative to admit and treat patients on their own. Thus the smaller figure should be used in any attempt to make the English admission privileges comparable to the American admission privileges.

family. As for the United States, it is erroneous to assume that only 23 percent of the physicians engage in providing so-called primary care. Because of the relative ease of initial access to specialists, the self-sorting of patients is not a tidy one as is the intent in England.[11] Although tidier than that of the United States, the Swedish system also permits some self-sorting of patients who can decide whether to see a general practitioner or a specialist for the initial visit during an illness episode. In Sweden, slightly over a third of all physicians are in private practice in their own offices. Unlike Britain, these are *not* all general practitioners but include some specialists who have no hospital appointments. In addition to the Swedish physicians who are totally in private practice, some hospital-based specialists practiced on a fee-for-service basis in the outpatient departments of polyclinics in the larger cities until the beginning of 1970. Counting these physicians as doing private practice brings the total up to about half of all Swedish physicians.

An appreciably higher proportion of physicians are listed as specialists in surgery in the United States than in Sweden or England. There are assumptions that there are more surgeons in the United States than are necessary for the current volume of surgical operations.[12] If that is true, it may be that surgeons are also providing other types of services. This is understandably true of general surgeons and those in rural areas. There is a well-founded assumption that all surgery in Sweden and England is performed by the American equivalent of Board Certified surgical specialists or under their supervision. In the United States in 1963, 54 percent of the surgery was performed by surgeons who were not Board Certified but had been given hospital privileges to perform operations on the basis of less formal criteria. This percentage has declined slightly from 1953, when 64 percent of all surgery was by non-Board Certified physicians.[13] In any case, evaluations of the quality of surgery performed in the three countries can hardly be precise.

The relatively small proportion of British physicians who are "medical specialists, 14 percent, compared with the United States and Sweden appears anomalous. It may be that the relatively large proportion of general practitioners results in a smaller portion of hospital-based "medical" specialists, especially pediatricians. It is also of interest that only 2 percent of the physician supply in England is engaged in administration compared with 7 and 9 percent in the United States and Sweden.

[11] It should also be noted that the United States classification is based on the physician's self-report and not actual certification as in the other two countries.
[12] Bunker (1970).
[13] Andersen and Anderson (1967), p. 33.

The number of active registered nurses also showed great variations between the three countries in 1950, with the United States being the highest by far. By 1968, Sweden had surpassed the United States, nearly doubling her registered nurse supply. The percentage increase in the other two countries was also substantial, as Table 10 shows. Still, all three countries complain about nursing shortages. Truly, there is no systematic knowledge regarding appropriate nursing staff ratios to patients or population.

TABLE 10   REGISTERED ACTIVE NURSES PER 100,000 POPULATION, 1950 and 1968

Country	1950	1968	Percent Increase
United States	249	331	33
Sweden	182	349	92
England	131	218	66

Source. Table A16.

Until Sweden increased the number of dentists in relation to population by 61 percent between 1950 and 1968, the United States had more dentists than any other Western country. In 1950, as seen in Table 11, the United States had 2½ times as many dentists as England and appreciably more than Sweden. Since 1950 the number of dentists in relation to population has remained virtually constant in both the United States and England, while Sweden increased the number of dentists per 100,-000 population from 49 to 79 in preparation for a universal dental care plan which has already been legislated but is yet to be inaugurated. It is of interest that England with a ratio of dentists to population considerably less than half of both the United States and Sweden has somehow man-

TABLE 11   DENTISTS PER 100,000 POPULATION, 1950 AND 1968

Country	1950	1968	Percent Increase
United States	57	57	—
Sweden	49	79	61
England	22	24	9

Source. Table A17.

aged to operate a universal dental plan since the inception of the National Health Service in 1948.

Among the various components of service, dental care seems to be the least open-ended. If the need of the population is fully met, there are only so many teeth to extract or fill or dentures to be fitted. There is very little of a psychosomatic nature here or of the perception of new diseases that is characteristic of diseases normally attended to by physicians in and out of the hospital. Hence the reservoir of dental need is relatively easy to measure. It is thus of great interest that there is much narrower variation among the number of physicians in the three countries than is true of dentists. There must, therefore, be an important difference in the volume of demand on the part of the population. It does not seem reasonable to assume that dentists in England are much more efficient than in the United States or Sweden and can hence handle a larger volume of service. Some evidence on use is presented in the following chapter.

VIII

The Use of Services

ALTHOUGH THERE ARE NOT systematic and long-term data on the use of services for all three countries, sufficiently detailed information is now available on the volume of use of the major components of services for current comparisons, particularly for hospital care. Routine information on physicians' services is not collected in any of the three countries. The United States has the best information on trends in the use of such services because of several nationwide household surveys that have been conducted since 1930. After a gap between 1930 and 1953, regular five-year surveys through 1963 were conducted by the Health Information Foundation and the National Opinion Research Center. Since 1960 the National Center for Health Statistics has also had surveys in this area and has published them in a series of reports.

The trend has been toward increased use in all three countries. At any given time however, there are differences between them. It is these differences, although the trends are the same, that intrigue researchers, administrators, and policy makers. In the early thirties in the United States the admission rate to general hospitals was about 60 per 1000 population with an average length of stay of 15 days, By 1970, the admission rate was 145 per 1,000 population and the average length of stay had dropped to 8 days.[1] In the early thirties approximately 40 percent of the popu-

[1] American Hospital Association (1971).

lation saw a physician at least once during a year, and the population as a whole experienced 2.5 visits per capita. Now the figures are 65 percent and about 4 respectively.

Sweden has parallel data on hospital use from the twenties but this is not available for physicians' services. England has neither. In the time frame from 1950 to the present time there are comparative social survey data on hospital use, but not on use of physicians' or dentists' services. Fortunately, however, there are current data from other sources on the use of physicians' and dentists' services for broad comparative purposes.

Although the number of hospital days of all types per 1000 population may be an incompatible case mix, it seems useful nevertheless to show how many days of hospital care in all hospitals (both short and long term) were utilized in the three systems in 1967. The United States experienced 2.5 days per person per year, Sweden 5, and England about 3. These would seem to be relatively large differences. Since 1950 there has been a moderate trend downward, due mainly to the rapid reduction in length of stay in mental hospitals and, to a smaller extent, tuberculosis hospitals. There have been only moderate changes in the general hospital days per 1000 population, except in the United States, as seen in Table 14.

TABLE 12   HOSPITAL DAYS PER 1000 POPULATION—
ALL HOSPITALS, 1968

Country	1968
United States	2524
Sweden	4957
England	2884

Source. Table A30.

TABLE 13   HOSPITAL DAYS PER 1000 POPULATION—
MENTAL HOSPITALS, 1960 AND 1968

Country	1960	1968
United States	1527	1082
Sweden	2329	2177
England	1606	1314

Source. Table A29.

TABLE 14   HOSPITAL DAYS PER 1000 POPULATION—
GENERAL HOSPITALS, 1950 AND 1968

Country	1950	1968
United States	890	1154
Sweden	1630	1569
England	1260[a]	1132

Source. Table A28.
[a]For 1960.

TABLE 15   ADMISSIONS TO GENERAL HOSPITALS PER 1000
POPULATION, 1950 AND 1968

Country	1950	1968	Percent Increase
United States	110	137	27
Sweden	113	138	22
England	64	98	53

Source. Table A25.

The number of admissions to general hospitals between 1950 and 1968, however, increased greatly, particularly in England. The length of stay has remained constant in the United States but has been reduced in Sweden and England which had a high of about 15 days a few years earlier. Other things being equal, one should expect the average length of stay to become shorter as the admission rate increases because of the increased

TABLE 16   AVERAGE LENGTH OF STAY—SHORT-TERM
GENERAL HOSPITALS 1950 AND 1968

Country	1950	1968
United States	8.1	8.4[b]
Sweden	15.8	11.9
England	15.0[a]	11.6

Source. Table A24.
[a] For 1960.
[b] An analysis of the year-by-year data shows a slight drop to 7.6 in 1960 and then an increase during the middle and late 1960s.

admission of less seriously ill patients. Yet in 1968 patients in Swedish hospitals had an average length of stay of almost 12 days compared with the United States average of 8 days even though the admission rates were similar.

For mental hospitals it appears that the same underlying forces are affecting the admission rate in all three countries: admissions are rising though the number of days per 1000 population is falling. Still, the relative differences in admission rates are tremendous, as seen in Table 17.

TABLE 17   ADMISSIONS TO MENTAL HOSPITALS PER 1000 POPULATION, 1950 AND 1968

Country	1950	1968
United States	3.2	4.6
Sweden	5.6[a]	11.0
England	1.4	4.1

Source. Table A26.
[a] For 1960.

The relative increase in Sweden is truly remarkable in view of the short time span, 1960 to 1967, for which data were obtainable. Sweden has doubled its admission rate to mental hospitals in seven years; the United States has increased its rate by 40 percent in 17 years and England has almost tripled its rate. Some of this increase is undoubtedly due to readmission of patients who previously would have remained hospitalized. Obviously, the care of mental illness is an exceedingly open-ended service.

In all three countries there is a great deal of concern and activity with mental day care centers to deemphasize institutional care and keep the patient in the community. In connection with mental hospitals all three countries experience great pressures for care of the aged who are incompetent and require custodial care but not the kind of care normally associated with mental hospitals. These are the ragged, undefined, and untidy edges of the patient care spectrum where the overlap between institutional acute care and community custodial care are difficult to define and cope with in any satisfactory manner.

Earlier comparisons have indicated that the United States and England are high in physician visits per person with about 5, and Sweden is low with about 3;[2] this picture may have been somewhat true in the past,

[2] Peterson et al., (1967), pp. 771–775.

though possibly distorted, but it is definitely not true today. The trend in the United States is toward somewhat *fewer* physician visits; most British figures cited have omitted outpatient consultations with specialists and have given only general practitioner figures. This is true of Peterson's pioneering work. Correcting for these two factors places the three countries along a continuum with England high at nearly 6 visits per person per year, the United States in the middle with about 4, and Sweden very low with only 2½. (See Table 18.) The Swedish figures are unfortunately seven years old, and with the increase in the physician-population ratio it is likely that the gap will have narrowed somewhat. It is also, of course, true that the Swedes take up some of the slack in their system with many more nurse visits than is true of the United States system; in fact, two sets of health practitioners in Sweden—the public health nurse who provides care (as opposed to supervision and planning) and the nurse-midwife—are virtually unknown in the United States. Even adding visits to nurses, however, would not take the total up to 4 visits per person per year.[3] It must be remembered too that England with its very high physician contact, also has fairly considerable services by nurses, especially midwives, which would further inflate its total. On the other hand, a good number of the English visits are in situations that do not involve medical care as such and would not result in visits in the United States and Sweden. These include renewal of prescriptions and certification of continuing disability, which must be done in person. All in all, the comparable English rate is probably somewhere between 5 and 6 visits per person per year with all adjustments made.

Other facets of health care use also emerge from Table 18. The percent of the population seeing a physician in a given year as determined by social survey is virtually the same in each of the countries—about two thirds. This is a remarkable finding in view of the very wide disparities in visits per person per year. What it means in effect is that *for people who go to the doctor at all in a given year* Swedes average 3.6 visits, Americans 6.3, and the British 8.9 visits. Evidently, the ease of initial contact is about the same in all three systems but, once in the system, factors are operating to cause the British to return for care more than twice as often as do the Swedes.

Considering the very high physician-contact rate in England, its somewhat higher average number of prescriptions filled per year is not surpris-

---

[3] Andersen, Smedby, and Anderson (1970) obtained figures of 3.99 visits for Sweden versus 5.47 for the United States for physician visits with all nurse visits included; Andersen's figures apply to the population 16 and over only. (Table 7, p. 18.)

TABLE 18 ANNUAL USE OF THE HEALTH CARE SYSTEM BY THE ENTIRE POPULATION

Country	Percent of Population Seeing a Physician	Average Number of Physician Visits per Year	Percent of Population Admitted to a General Hospital	Percent Using Prescribed Drugs	Average Number of Prescriptions Filled	Percent of Population Seeing a Dentist	Average Number of Dentist Visits per Year
United States	68	4.3	10.0	43	4.7	38	1.4
Sweden	69	2.5	8.5	62	4.5	43[b]	—
England	66	5.9	6.6[a]	46	5.8	37[b]	0.4[c]

Source. Table A31.
[a]Calculated by finding the ratio of single admissions to all admissions for the United States (0.73) and Sweden (0.65) and applying the midpoint (0.69) to all admissions for England.
[b]Excludes children under 16.
[c]Courses of treatment; actual number of dental visits was probably somewhat higher.

134

ing. What is of interest is the higher percent of the population using prescribed drugs in Sweden as compared to the United States or England; this may be an artifact of the statistics, however.[4]

About the same percentage of people see a dentist in the United States and England; the slightly higher figure in the table for Sweden would be somewhat higher still if children, with their higher average number of visits, could be added. We saw earlier that the Swedes had the highest dentist-population ratio of the three countries and was, moreover, the only one with an increasing dentist-population ratio over the years. The most sketchy of the data shown in the table relate to the average number of dental visits per year. It is almost certain that the English figure is understated but it is almost equally certain that, could a comparable figure be obtained, it would still be lower than the American. One bit of evidence on this is that the percentage of the adult population without any

CHART 1   COMPARATIVE PERSONNEL AND UTILIZATION
IN THE THREE COUNTRIES, 1967

Aspect of Utilization	United States	Sweden	England
Physicians per 1000 population	High	Low	Low
Average number of physician visits per year	Medium	Low	High
Percent of population seeing a physician	Same	Same	Same
General hospital admissions per 1000 population	High	High	Low
Length of stay	Low	High	High
General hospital days per 1000 population	Medium	High	Medium
Dentists per 1000 population	Medium	High	Low
Percent of population seeing a dentist	Same	Same	Same
Prescriptions filled per person	Low	Low	High

[4] Eight percent of the Swedish population said they had not had a prescription filled during a household interview but a prescription was found for them when drug records were verified. (Andersen, Smedby, and Anderson (1970), p. 146.) This crosschecking was not possible in the U.S. or Great Britain. Subtracting this eight percent still leaves Sweden with a rather high usage, however.

natural teeth is 37 percent in England but only 18 percent in the United States.[5] Were the Swedish figure on dental visits available, it would undoubtedly be the highest of all.[6]

In summary, the three systems are fairly similar on some aspects of their utilization but very different on others (Chart 1).

There are no easy generalizations about the three systems. With all the complicating details in mind, however, it can be said that Swden tends to provide its medical care on an inpatient basis while England relies much more on outpatient treatment. The United States is midway between the two more "socialized" systems on this dimension. Without an elaborately developed and generally agreed upon weighting system for all facets of health care, it is impossible to say which country does the most for its citizens.

[5] Department of Health and Social Security (1970).
[6] Swedish dental care is a conglomeration of private dental treatment, public treatment without charge for all children, and some public treatment for adults who either are poor or live in inaccessible spots.

IX

Trends in Expenditures

Previous chapters have shown increases in personnel and use which, of course, add up to increased expenditures. There has also been an increase in the income of health care personnel, particularly for the lower and nonprofessional grades, relative to the wage levels of the rest of the labor market. Another factor, difficult to measure with current data but undoubtedly present, is the increase in various types of medical technology in the form of complex equipment and chemotherapy and its associated personnel.

Table 19 shows that the increase in expenditures both for the total population and per capita from 1950 to 1968 was by far the greatest for

TABLE 19 PERCENT INCREASE IN EXPENDITURES FOR THE
HEALTH SERVICES FROM 1950 TO 1968

Country	Total Population	Per Capita
United States	320	221
Sweden	1043	912
England	219	159

Source. Table A4.

137

Sweden followed by the United States and England. The more comparable of the two measures is the per capita increase because of the relatively
large growth in the United States population during that period.

The economies of the three countries have also been very active as seen
by the gross measure of national income (Table 20). Even accounting for
inflation as measured by the consumer price indices in the three countries, the increases in national income have been substantial. In the
United States there was an increase in the consumer price index from
1950 to 1969 of 52 percent, in Sweden 119 percent, and in England 91
percent.

TABLE 20   PERCENT INCREASE IN NATIONAL INCOME
FROM 1950 TO 1968

Country	National Income
United States	220
Sweden	377
England	203

Source. Table A7.

Although all three countries had substantial absolute increases in their
national incomes, they allotted variable proportions of their national incomes to health services and at differential rates of increase. Table 21
shows that the rank order of expenditures as a percent of gross national
income had the United States and England about the same in 1950 with
Sweden considerably lower. By 1968 this relationship had been virtually
reversed with Sweden the highest, closely followed by the United States,
and England the lowest. By 1970, the U.S. had increased its health care
expenditures as a percent of national income to 8.4 and England to 5.6.

TABLE 21   TOTAL COST OF THE HEALTH SERVICES AS A
PERCENT OF NATIONAL INCOME, 1950 TO 1968

Country	1950	1968
United States	5.3	7.5
Sweden	3.2	8.1
England	5.4	5.2

Source. Table A6.

Comparable figures for Sweden are unavailable.

For the 18 year period for which data are available for all three countries, Sweden has more than doubled its proportion of national income spent for health care, the U.S. has increased its proportion by about 40 percent, and the English percentage has actually decreased slightly. Thus the United States falls midway between the two more "socialized" systems in its increase in health care expenditures using the most comparative measure possible. There is, then, no clear relationship between extent of governmental control of the health care system and control of health care costs.

In overall economic productivity the three countries were not on the same level in 1950 nor are they today. In 1950 both the United States and England were allocating about the same proportion of gross national income for their respective health services, that is, somewhat over 5 percent. Since the United States gross income was and is considerably larger per capita than that of England, the United States obviously spent in absolute terms more per person on its health services than England and thus starts at a higher absolute base for comparisons 18 years later. Sweden spent only 3.2 percent of its gross national income in 1950 on health services; its per capita gross national income was not as high as that of the United States but higher than that of England. Eighteen years later Sweden clearly exceeds the expenditure level of England and has indeed surpassed that of the United States.

Compared to consumer price index increases, in 1968 Sweden had increased its expenditures for health services nine times as rapidly, the United States seven times as rapidly, and England two and a half times as rapidly.[1] Expenditures for health services increased 2.8 times as fast as national income in Sweden and 1.5 times as fast in the United States. In England, national income and health care expenditures increased at about the same rate.

The foregoing data have dealt with total health service expenditures. A previous chapter showed the distribution of the medical dollar by components of services. In data to follow, the trends in expenditures will be broken out by selected components to show movements between them.

Table 22 has been standardized because of the widely varying inflation and consequent unequal rate of increase for health care services in the

---

[1] Of course the expenditure increases for health services is made up of three components: (1) population increase; (2) increased use per person; (3) price per unit increase. The clear tendency, however, has been for the health service prices to increase faster than general prices. There is currently no way to compare prices for health services between the three countries.

TABLE 22   INCREASES IN PER CAPITA EXPENDITURES FOR
SELECTED HEALTH SERVICE COMPONENTS RELATED TO TOTAL
RATE OF INCREASE FROM 1950 TO 1965

Country	Hospital	Physician	Dentist	Drugs	Nursing Homes	All Services
United States	106	84	68	69	525	100
Sweden	79	79	109	104	121	100
England	76	59	32	122	73	100

Source. Derived from Tables A4 and A8.

three countries. Using the rate of increase for total services as a base, it can be seen that nursing homes and hospitals accounted for the greatest increase in the United States, nursing homes and dentists in Sweden, and drugs in England.

In concluding our discussion of cost trends, it is important to point out that during the period under discussion, the only country that had anything approaching a national policy for its health services was England, and even there it was not explicit. England has been emphasizing equality of access since 1948 and has an administrative structure aimed at carrying out this mandate. Obviously, England had made this attempt at less cost than either Sweden or the United States.

X

The Payoff—Health Levels, Accessibility, and Family Solvency

W E HAVE SEEN PATTERNS of personnel, funding, and trends in use among the three countries that are very difficult to explain. This chapter will make clear that it is difficult to show direct relationship of the foregoing elements to the usual health indices of morbidity and mortality. And these indices are popularly assumed to have a rather direct relationship to the inputs of a health service of an area. Indeed, it is difficult not to assume otherwise because policy makers and administrators have to believe there is a health payoff for the enormous resources that countries are now putting into their health services.

The only way to find out what influence health services by themselves have on the health indices is to withdraw all personal health services from a test population which had a good standard of living, adequate incomes, pure air, wholesome working conditions, good diets, moderate habits—and measure the usual health indices in the absence of personal health services. It is unlikely that the death rate would rise appreciably, because in all three countries there has been a diminishing margin of deaths that can be prevented by known means even if fully applied. What the future holds in the prevention and cure of heart disease, cancer, and stroke is another question. Some years ago estimates were made as to the causes of death that could actually be eliminated given current knowledge. For the United States it was estimated that there could be a mortality reduction of only around 6 percent given the full application of current medical diagnosis and treatment.[1] Changes in life styles affecting diet, smoking, and exercise would have an appreciable effect in reducing mortality according to well-formulated studies, but the changing of life styles is not a medical responsibility in the technical sense of the word.[2] As Dubos somewhat despairingly but truthfully wrote some years ago:

> In the words of a wise physician, it is part of the doctor's function to make it possible for his patients to go on doing the pleasant things that are bad for them—smoking too much, eating too much, drinking too much—without killing themselves any sooner than is necessary.[3]

Comparative health indices will be given detailed attention in order to put the vital statistical international race into some perspective. Perhaps the United States can be better motivated to improve its health indices in relation to other developed nations by engaging in an international health indices race à la Sputnik. The United States might then learn that neither the methods to accomplish this nor the results of the efforts are as clearly measured as a race to the moon.

On the other hand, it is too extreme a position to denigrate the current importance that personal health services per se have on health indices. Obviously *public* health measures have had a demonstrable effect on death rates from cholera, typhoid, smallpox, poliomyelitis, and malaria,—measures that can be carried out without a personal health service apparatus, as is commonly done in developing countries. It can further be assumed that a truly tremendous increase in the resources of personal health services such as those provided for politicians, presidents, prime ministers, or an exceedingly rich citizen would have a demonstrable effect on length of life.

[1] Anderson and Lerner (1960), p. 30.

[2] A recent study of the relationship between the mortality of whites and both medical care and environmental variables suggests that environmental variables are far more important than medical care. High income is associated with high mortality when medical care and education are controlled for. The study observes: "This may reflect unfavorable diets, lack of exercise, psychological tensions, etc. The positive association of mortality with income may explain the failure of death rates to decline rapidly in recent years" (Auster, Leveson, and Sarachek). Of course, studies that consider the relationship of mortality to income without controlling for medical care and education show an opposite relationship.

[3] Dubos (1959), pp. 179–180.

It is doubtful however, that any country is willing to allocate, either privately or publicly, as great a portion of its national income as a saturation-type health service would require. Short of this objective, a steadily increasing allocation of resources to the health services will be assumed as long as medical technology continues to develop and as unmet need remains, however defined from simple care to protracted rehabilitation. The yardstick of achievement, however, cannot be the mortality rate alone; other indices need to be brought in. One of them is the alleviation of anxiety by the very presence of personal health services. Another is how far the ideal of access to health services as a civil right has been realized. Hence, we discuss here these yardsticks of achievements as well as the health indices.

Most of the discussions of the relative merits and demerits of the three systems have been in general terms using fragmentary, sometimes quite old, data which are frequently not comparable. In the last few years, more specific, carefully researched articles and books have begun to appear [4] but most of these have concentrated primarily on utilization and its specific relationship to the structural differences of the three systems. Although utilization itself has sometimes been considered the "product" of a health care system, in actuality it is the *result* of utilization that is the product.

There is as yet no general agreement on what this result or outcome should be called. This does not mean that the topic has been neglected by the health care field but rather that it is so extremely complicated and many-faceted that advocates of the different disciplines have come up with varying, sometimes contradictory, measures of outcome. These can be best summed up under two headings: satisfaction of the patient, which may include psychic comfort as well as physical well-being or relative relief, and physical effect on the patient, which includes the well-known demographic variables of mortality, morbidity, and disability. Satisfaction of the patient is becoming increasingly more important, as fewer and fewer contacts between the patient and the health care system are a matter of life and death. Unfortunately studies of patient satisfaction are only now beginning to appear while the concept of actual physical effects has been around for a long time and is embodied in the familiar and at least superficially comparable concept of vital statistics which are measurable in concrete terms. Mortality is the most specific—and final—of these vital statistics. Since mortality is dependent to a great extent on the demographic characteristics of a given country, independent of the influ-

[4] Bunker (1970), Peterson, et al., (1967); Andersen, Smedby, and Anderson (1970); Fry (1970).

ence of the health care system, population differences are intertwined to such an extent that they deserve brief mention here, in addition to the geographical dimensions that were presented earlier.

POPULATION DIFFERENCES

In addition to geographical differences other, more subtle, characteristics of the population greatly affect the demand on the health services and the type of utilization they will be subject to. The United States has long had the highest birth rate of the three countries; it is only in the last few years that it has fallen close to that of England and Sweden. While Sweden and England experienced only a moderate rise in their birth rates during the 1950s, the United States had a full scale baby boom then, as

TABLE 23   BIRTH RATE PER 1000 POPULATION

| Year | United States | | | Sweden | England |
	White	Nonwhite	Total		
1935	17.9	25.8	18.8	13.8	14.8
1945	19.7	26.5	20.8	20.2	18.3
1950	23.0	33.3	24.5	16.5	15.8
1955	23.8	34.7	25.3	14.8	15.0
1960	22.7	32.1	23.9	13.7	17.1
1965	18.3	27.6	19.4	15.9	18.1
1966	17.4	26.1	18.4	15.8	17.7
1967	16.8	25.0	17.8	15.4	17.2
1968	16.6	24.2	17.5	14.2	16.9

Sources. United States: Bureau of the Census (1968), pp. 47–48; NCHS, *Monthly Vital Statistics Report,* Vol. 18, No. 11. Sweden: National Board of Health (1971), p. 149. England: Department of Health and Social Security (1969), p. 77.

Table 23 shows. The babies born are coming to maturity now, shifting the age structure of the United States more toward the childbearing years and inevitably forcing up the total number of births and the birth rate. As of 1971, however, this has not yet occurred, and the total U.S. birth rate is at almost an all-time low—about 15.0.

Thus, other things being equal, the health care system in the United

States has been required to provide more prenatal care, deliveries, post-natal care, and infant preventive care than are systems in the other two countries. Also in the United States the nonwhite birth rate has always been substantially higher than the white rate; the white rate has, in fact, since 1965 been lower than in England. Since the nonwhite population in the United States is considerably less well-educated and has much lower incomes than the white population, a substantial load must be assumed by the United States health care system for these births in addition to the extra care required by its unusually high birth rate in general.

Besides the problems posed by the high birth rate among the lower socioeconomic segments of the population, a problem shared by England and Sweden though not nearly to the same extent, the United States is faced with the problem of illegitimacy among the same population. Illegitimate births are more likely to be complicated by poor motivation to seek prenatal care and inadequate care of the newborn child, both factors that make the job of the health care system more difficult. As Table 24 shows, the United States actually has a smaller percentage of illegitimate births overall than does Sweden and only slightly higher than does England, but these illegitimate births are concentrated among the nonwhite segment of the population, a group that is already less likely to receive prenatal care and less likely to have a good environment for the infant.

Other differences in the population of the three countries have to do with the early age at marriage and childbearing in the United States. Nearly 15 percent of the United States births take place before the age of 20, a relatively unfavorable time for childbearing, both physically and economically, compared with 11 percent of the Swedish births and 8 per-

TABLE 24   PERCENT OF BIRTHS WHICH ARE ILLEGITIMATE

Year	United States			Sweden	England
	White	Nonwhite	Total		
1950	1.7	18.0	4.0	9.8	4.9
1960	2.3	21.6	5.3	11.3	5.8
1966	4.4	27.6	8.4	14.6	7.7
1968	5.3	31.2	9.7	15.1	8.4

Sources. United States: Bureau of Census (1971), p. 49. Sweden: 1950 from NCHS, Series 3, No. 6 (1967), p. 69; 1960, 1966 and 1968 from National Central Bureau of Statistics (1970), p. 76. England: Central Statistical Office (1970), p. 56.

cent of the British births. The higher United States birthrate has also resulted in a greater number of births to women of high parity and, again, these births carry with them an added risk. Although these factors need to be taken into account, their effect on *overall* mortality is rather small, since in all three countries the majority of the births occur at favorable ages and parities. These factors are most important in populations where a substantial number of the births occur at very young ages or high parity, as among Negroes in the United States.

Finally, the attitudes toward legal abortions vary greatly in the three countries. Sweden has long had the most liberal law and in 1968 was terminating one pregnancy for every 10 live births. Since the law concentrates on physical problems in the mother, possible defects in the child, mothers of high parity or of very young age, and mothers with social problems, it is obvious that the tendency is to terminate high-risk pregnancies. The British law was previously rather restrictive so that, as late as 1965, only one in every 200 pregnancies was legally aborted; at present, under a new and revised law, the British are aborting about one pregnancy for every 10 live births. The United States has long had the most restrictive abortion laws on a state-by-state basis and in 1966 was aborting only one out of every 2000 pregnancies legally; the situation had changed by 1969 to one abortion for every 170 live births and in 1971 to one abortion for every 7 live births.

In the United States, before legalised abortion, it was estimated that there was one illegal abortion for every four live births. Unlike Sweden where problem pregnancies likely to have a high mortality rate are terminated, the situation in the United States favored illegal abortion of healthy, well-educated women. The recent changes in the laws in all three countries will undoubtedly serve to bring about a convergence in the type of pregnancies being terminated.

These distinctions among the populations of the three countries have been discussed in detail because the populations are so different that the health outcomes would necessarily be different even if the health systems were identical. In particular, the details surrounding the differences in how pregnancy is handled in the three countries are crucial to an understanding of why infant mortality rates vary so much. Clearly, because of tradition and social problems, the United States health care system has had more to overcome than the other two systems. Whether it does as well as can be expected under the circumstances is a separate and legitimate question.

MORTALITY DIFFERENCES

It was stated earlier that the outcome of utilization of the health care system could be measured in two major ways: satisfaction or comfort of the patient and actual physical changes, as measured by morbidity, disability, and mortality. This subject is so complex that an entire book could be written on it alone. Suffice it to say that there are virtually no comparative data on satisfaction and comfort, and therefore we must fall back upon the more conventional and somewhat limited demographic information. The rest of this chapter is concerned only with mortality. In passing it should be noted that morbidity and disability statistics are in some ways inversely related to mortality statistics; when mortality is low, morbidity can sometimes be high. An example of this is that strenuous efforts to save babies born with serious congenital defects will decrease the infant mortality rate while at the same time increasing the morbidity and disability rates for young children.

A basic assumption in comparing mortality in the three countries is that social conditions, level of subsistence, customs, and level of susceptibility to illness are similar in the populations so that any differences that might occur are the result of differing effectiveness of the health care systems. It has already been seen that this assumption is not accurate in the case of social conditions surrounding pregnancy and birth in the three countries. The United States system could not produce as favorable an infant mortality rate as the other two countries even if its health care system were identical to theirs. It is equally obvious that the same variables affect other aspects of mortality as well so that the mortality comparisons that will now be made do not reflect the inferiority or superiority of any of the systems but rather a measure of how well each system does, *given the social and cultural conditions and priorities it has to work with.* A health service cannot be expected to compensate for the deleterious effects on health of a social system.

With these cautions in mind, let us look at the most common mortality indices. The most often mentioned and the one that shows the most difference among countries is the infant mortality rate. Here the United States has been severely criticized for what is regarded as "preventable" deaths and for not applying its technology to the fullest.

It should be noted first that, while England and Sweden have sometimes been lumped together in those countries which are "superior" to the United States in this regard, the English rate is actually rather similar to the United States one while the Swedish rate is markedly lower than either. Since 1950 the English and Swedish rates have been declining more rapidly than the United States rate: 42 percent for Great Britain, 38 percent for Sweden, but only 25 percent for the United States and, within the United States, only 23 percent for the nonwhite population. Thus the United States is in the position of having very high infant mortality rates coupled with a slower rate of improvement than those in the other two countries.

TABLE 25   INFANT MORTALITY RATES

	United States				
Year	White	Nonwhite	Total	Sweden	England
1950	26.8	44.5	29.2	21.0	31.4
1960	22.9	43.2	26.0	16.6	21.8
1965	21.5	40.3	24.7	13.3	19.0
1967	19.7	35.9	22.1	12.9	18.4
1968	19.2	34.5	21.8	13.0	18.3
1969	a	a	20.7	a	18.0

Sources. United States: Bureau of the Census (1971), p. 55. Sweden: National Board of Health (1971), p. 149. England: 1950 calculated from Central Statistical Office (1965); 1960–1967 from Department of Health and Social Security Digest (1969), p. 1; 1968–1969 from ibid (1971), p. 2.

Many of the reasons for this were discussed earlier, either overtly or by implication. One of the most important factors, which operated until very recently was the much higher United States birth rate, concentrated among lower-income groups and coupled with a very restrictive abortion policy and difficulties in obtaining regular and effective birth control information. It can be argued that the very difficult social problems among many of the disadvantaged American groups may create an "excess" postneonatal mortality that even superhuman efforts of the health care system cannot entirely alleviate. In this connection, it should be noted that the United States and English postneonatal mortality rates are identical, suggesting the operation of many of the same social forces in that country as in the United States.

Even though the heterogeneous United States with social conditions favoring a higher birth rate is unlikely to achieve the same low level of infant mortality as homogeneous, more tightly controlled Sweden, it is nevertheless undoubtedly true that part of the deficit must be laid at the doorstep of the health care system itself. It will be seen later that Sweden,

TABLE 26 SELECTED INDICES RELATED TO
INFANT MORTALITY

Country and Year	Birthrate per 1000 Population	Fetal Mortality per 1000 Total Births	Infant Mortality per 1000 Live Births		
			Under 1 Year	Under 28 Days	28 Days to 11 Months
United States, 1967	17.8	15.0	22.1	16.2	5.9
Sweden, 1968	14.2	9.4	13.0	10.5	2.5
England, 1968	16.9	10.1	18.3	12.4	5.9

Sources. United States: Bureau of the Census (1968), pp. 47–55. Breakdown of infant mortality from NCHS, *Monthly Vital Statistics Report,* Vol. 17, No. 12, 1969. Sweden: National Central Bureau of Statistics (1970), pp. 76–77. England: Department of Health and Social Security (1969), pp. 77, 100.

at least, tends to concentrate its resources on babies, children, and young adults to a greater extent than does the United States, which concentrates more of its resources on old people.[5] It is also undoubtedly true that the easier provision of birth control information, and concentration of legal abortions on high-risk babies rather than illegal abortions on the babies of well-off mothers, are just as much facets of the health care system as is the actual provision of prenatal care and delivery. In this connection, the United States maternal mortality rate was, in 1966, 2.9 per 10,000 live births (and a phenomenally high 7.2 for nonwhite mothers) compared with 2.6 for England and only 1.1 for Sweden. A large percent of the United States and English rates were, at that time, made up of the after-effects of illegal abortions,[6] a negligible problem in Sweden.

Even so, it appears to be true that prenatal care and deliveries are much less uniformly provided in the United States, where they are an individual contract between patient and physician with public facilities fragmentary and restricted to those who cannot pay. Such services are

[5] Andersen, Smedby, and Anderson (1970), pp. 43–45, 46, 48–49.
[6] In the United States in 1967, 23 percent of the complications of maternal deaths for which a cause was given were due to abortion [NCHS (1969), calculated from p. 1–40]. In Britain in 1966, 23 percent of all maternal deaths were due to abortion, with three quarters of the abortions specified as illegal [Department of Health and Social Security (1969), pp. 81–82.]

more uniformly provided in England and Sweden. As Table 26 has shown, it is actually in the areas of fetal mortality and early infant mortality that the United States has the worst record relative to the other two countries. These two areas would undoubtedly benefit from more coordinated, easily accessible care. Even in England and Sweden a class differential remains in infant mortality though it is not as large as in the United States,[7] thus underscoring the importance of other factors even when the health care system is ostensibly the same for all.

Let us turn now to age-specific mortality throughout the life span and see how the three countries fare. It is apparent that in the United States people with fatal illnesses put a smaller burden on the health care system than they do in either England or Sweden; 9.4 Americans out of every 1000 die in a year compared with 10.1 in Sweden and 11.1 in Great Britain. This is, of course, due to the younger age of the United States population and not to any intrinsic healthiness or superior medical care. In fact, looking at mortality by age group, the pattern emerges that the United States has many more deaths in infancy, does about the same as the other two countries in childhood, has more deaths in the productive years of adulthood, and has fewer deaths than either country in extreme old age. Comparing England and Sweden, the rates are quite similar throughout but the Swedish experience is very slightly better at nearly every age and considerably better in infancy. Rates for all age groups in all three countries have undergone some slight improvement since 1965 but far less than in previous time periods.

Table 27 tends to confirm a supposition previously mentioned—the United States system concentrates on care for the elderly relative to children while the British and Swedish systems do the reverse. This is, however, not the only interpretation of the data: it is a generally recognized phenomenon in demography that groups with relatively poor health experiences and very high death rates in childhood and early adulthood frequently show very low mortality in extreme old age. For instance, Albania and Greece, two countries with rather poor early mortality rates, have the lowest rates recorded over 65.[8] It will be seen that this is true of the American Black population as well. So it is quite possible that the excellent showing of the United States in the oldest age groups is not due to additional health care lavished on the elderly but merely to the fact that those who get to be elderly are an exceptionally healthy and tenacious lot. The question is certainly still open. In any case, it is difficult to establish precise ages in any country in the upper-age limits.

[7] NCHS, Series 3, No. 6, pp. 67–69.
[8] United Nations (1968), pp. 420–424.

TABLE 27 AGE-SPECIFIC MORTALITY, 1965

	Deaths per 1000 Population		
Age	United States	Sweden	England
Under 1	24.1	13.3	20.5
1–4	0.9	0.7	0.8
5–14	0.4	0.4	0.4
15–24	1.1	0.7	0.8
25–34	1.5	1.0	0.9
35–44	3.1	1.9	2.1
45–54	7.4	4.4	5.8
55–64	16.9	11.3	15.1
65–74	37.9	32.3	32.0
75 and over	101.7	110.9	111.1
Overall	9.4	10.1	11.1

Sources. United States: Bureau of the Census (1968), p. 55. Sweden: National Central Bureau of Statistics (1968), p. 78. England: Central Statistical Office (1965), p. 27. Calculated by weighting for the ratio of males to females at each age level from p. 8. Death rates for ages 1 to 4 taken from Department of Health and Social Security (1969), p. 100. All data are for United Kingdom for 1964.

Why is the United States mortality higher than that of Sweden and England at most age levels? It has sometimes been maintained that the differential is due to the extremely poor health record of Blacks, but a glance at Table 28 shows that even with the Black mortality eliminated, the United States rates are still not as low as those of Sweden at most age levels.

Table 28 also makes an important point that is very frequently overlooked: although the differential between white and nonwhite infant mortality is the one most noticed in the literature, the greatest differential in mortality actually occurs in the adult years of 25 to 44 when the Black rate is more than 2½ times the white rate. Deaths from homicide, drug addiction, accidents, concomitants of alcoholism, and other causes reflective more of social problems than of specific failings in the health care system take their toll here. However, the differential is probably too great to be explained by social conditions and undoubtedly reflects an actual difference in available care. It will be noted that the Black and white death rates are the same overall, but this is of course due to the greatly younger age of the Black population.

TABLE 28   AGE-SPECIFIC MORTALITY BY COLOR—
UNITED STATES, 1967

Age	Deaths per 1000 Population		
	White	Nonwhite	Total
Under 1	19.6	35.4	22.3
1–4	0.8	1.4	0.9
5–14	0.4	0.6	0.4
15–24	1.1	1.7	1.2
25–34	1.3	3.5	1.5
35–44	2.7	6.7	3.1
45–54	6.7	12.9	7.3
55–64	15.9	25.5	16.7
65–74	36.1	53.7	37.5
75–84	80.0	67.3	79.0
85 and over	203.8	108.5	194.2
Overall	9.4	9.4	9.4

Source. National Center for Health Statistics, *Vital Statistics* (1969), Vol. II–A, pp. 1–4.

A subject to which justice cannot be done in this book is that of cause-specific mortality. Suffice it to say that the leading causes of death are very similar in all three countries and in the United States rather similar between white and nonwhite. The main variations from the prevailing United States pattern occur in the high rate due to homicide among nonwhites, deaths due to bronchitis in England, and the high Swedish suicide rate, which is currently about twice that of the United States and England.

It would seem that a crude though significant measure of health levels is the rank order of causes of mortality as presented in Table 29. When a country or social class within a country attains the status of heart disease being the leading cause of death followed by cancer, stroke, and accidents, obviously profound social and medical transformations have taken place in that the controllable scourges of the past have been displaced as the leading causes of death. Everything else being equal, the greater the proportion of deaths that can be attributed to heart disease, the greater has been the impact of environing factors that affect differentials in causes of death at young age levels. Indeed, it appears that Sweden's mortality rate due to heart disease is greater than that of either the United States or England. This seems reasonable when one examines the extent

TABLE 29   TEN LEADING CAUSES OF DEATH—UNITED STATES,
SWEDEN, ENGLAND AND WALES, LATE 1960'S

United States			
White	Nonwhite	Sweden	England and Wales
(1) Heart disease	Heart disease	Heart disease	Heart disease
(2) Cancer	Cancer	Cancer	Cancer
(3) Stroke	Stroke	Stroke	Stroke
(4) Accidents	Accidents	Influenza and pneumonia	Influenza and pneumonia
(5) Influenza and pneumonia	Diseases of early infancy	Accidents	Bronchitis
(6) Diseases of early infancy	Influenza and pneumonia	Hypertension	Accidents
(7) Hypertension	Homicide	Suicide	General arteriosclerosis
(8) General arteriosclerosis	Diabetes	Diabetes	Hypertension
(9) Diabetes	General arteriosclerosis	Diseases of early infancy	Diseases of early infancy
(10) Suicide	Hypertension	Senility	Suicide

Sources. United States: National Center for Health Statistics, *Vital Statistics,*
Vol. II–B (1969), pp. 7–14 to 7–127. Sweden: National Central Bureau of Statis-
tics (1968), pp. 289–291. England and Wales: Derived from Central Statistical
Office (1965), p. 33.

to which the three countries approximate a theoretical level of attainment.

In order to show the theoretical level of attainment, it was decided to
use the lowest age-specific mortality rate reported for any one age group
in any country reporting in a recent United Nations Demographic Yearbook as the possible level of attainment. Such a level of attainment is
really more than theoretical because it exists. So, then, instead the United
States, Sweden, and England being compared with one another, they are
compared with a worldwide level of attainment as experienced by a composite of age groups from all the reporting countries of the world. The
following differences emerge: Sweden reveals exceedingly good levels of
attainment in the younger age groups but less so in the upper groups
when death has to take its toll at some time anyway. It is theoretically

impossible for a country to have the lowest death rates in the world for all age groups. High survival in the younger age groups must result in higher death rates in the upper age groups as long as the leading causes of death in the upper age groups cannot be controlled in any large-scale sense by medical means.

The Swedish (and other Scandinavian) mortality rates continue to be intriguing to students of the health services. To pursue this interest further the states with the lowest mortality rates in the United States plus Minnesota were selected. The state that proved to have the lowest rate in

CHART 2   THE LOWEST AGE-SPECIFIC DEATH RATES RECORDED IN WESTERN COUNTRIES, LATE 1960s

Age	Country with Lowest Rate	Rate[a]
Under 1	Sweden	12.7
1– 4	Sweden	0.7
5– 9	Belgium, Denmark, France, Hungary, Sweden, Great Britain, Scotland, Australia, New Zealand, United States	0.4
10–14	Denmark, France, Hungary, Sweden, Great Britain	0.3
15–19	Ireland	0.5
20–24	Denmark, Netherlands, Norway, Great Britain	0.7
25–29	Netherlands, Sweden	0.7
30–34	Norway, Sweden, Great Britain	1.0
35–39	Greece, Netherlands	1.3
40–44	Greece	2.1
45–49	Greece, Sweden	3.3
50–54	Greece	5.1
55–59	Greece, Sweden	8.2
60–64	Greece	13.4
65–69	Norway	23.2
70–74	Greece	36.4
75–79	Albania	59.1
80–84	Albania	75.8
85 and over	Albania	107.0

Source. United Nations (1968), pp. 420–425.

[a]Excludes countries with less than one million population because of the small number of deaths in some age categories. If it were not for this exclusion Iceland would have the lowest death rate in six categories and the Island of Malta in an additional four categories.

CHART 3 PERCENT ATTAINMENT OF OPTIMUM AGE-SPECIFIC
MORTALITY RATES–UNITED STATES, 1966

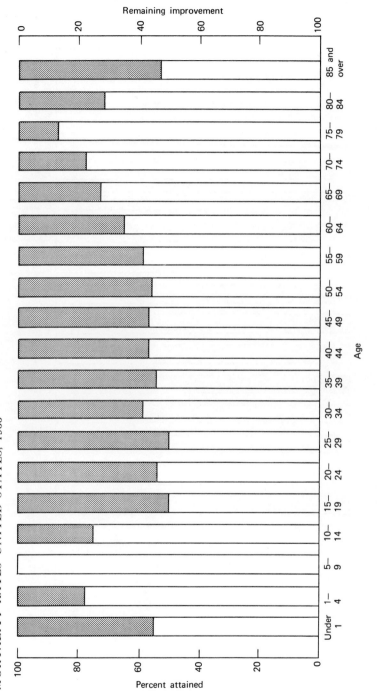

155

CHART 4 PERCENT ATTAINMENT OF OPTIMUM AGE-SPECIFIC
MORTALITY RATES—SWEDEN, 1966

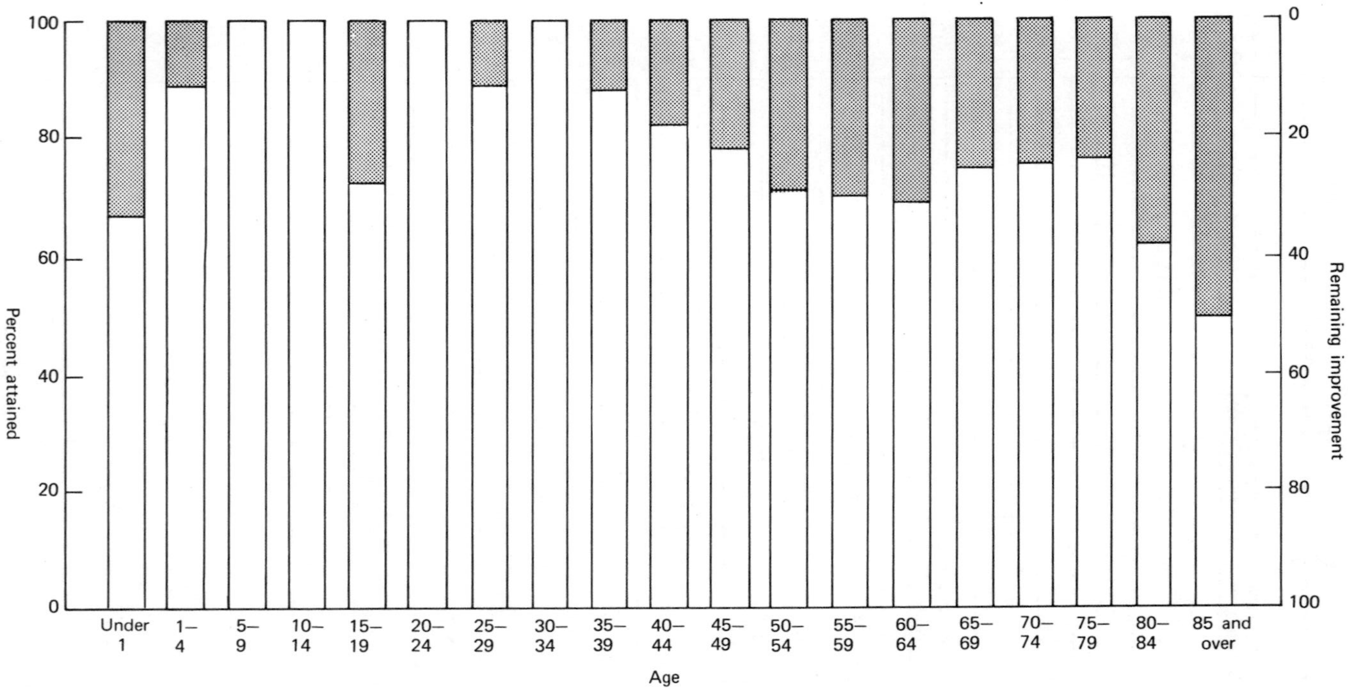

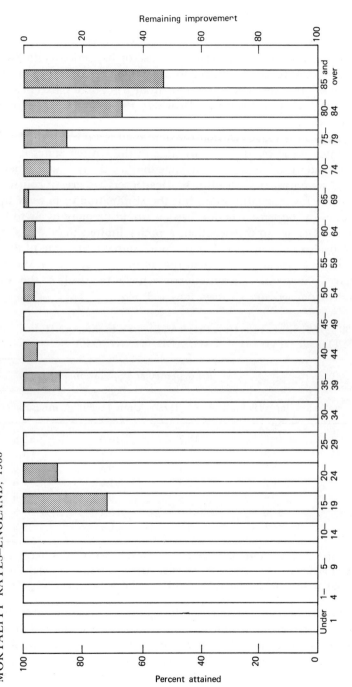

CHART 5 PERCENT ATTAINMENT OF OPTIMUM AGE-SPECIFIC MORTALITY RATES—ENGLAND, 1966

all age groups (with the exception of the infant mortality rate which was so close as to render the difference meaningless) was Hawaii, with Utah a close second. Minnesota was selected because of its similarity to Sweden in climate, economy, and a population of Northern European stock. Table 30 shows that Sweden is lower than all three states, except for the age group 65 and over (and 5 to 19 where the difference is extremely small in any case).

The conclusion is suggested that the dominant reason why the Swedish mortality rates are lower than in any state in the United States is a high minimum standard of living for everyone and a cultural homogeneity of life styles of sanitation and cleanliness. Health services are, of course, also a factor in the low mortality rates, but the elimination of poverty in the United States in the sense true for Sweden would be more likely to bring mortality rates closer to Sweden than a policy limited to health services only. It can also be ventured that the predominant life style of Sweden results in more physical activity than that of the United States. When the Swedes have as many private automotive vehicles relatively as the Americans, deaths from sedentary causes may well rise.

TABLE 30   AGE-SPECIFIC DEATH RATES—SWEDEN, AND THE STATES OF HAWAII, UTAH, AND MINNESOTA

Age	Rate per 1000 Population			
	Sweden (1968)	Hawaii (1969)	Utah (1969)	Minnesota (1969)
Under 1	12.9	16.7	16.6	19.8
Under 5	3.2	3.7	4.1	4.1
5–19	0.5	0.4	0.5	0.6
20–44	1.2	1.5	1.6	1.6
45–64	7.4	8.3	9.0	9.6
65 and over	57.6	51.0	55.4	56.3
All ages	10.1	5.2	6.4	9.2

Sources. United States: National Center for Health Statistics, *Vital Statistics,* Vol. II–A (1969), pp. 1–31 and 2–6. Sweden: Derived from National Board of Health (1969), p. 152, and National Central Bureau of Statistics (1968), p. 78.

It can hardly be claimed that the foregoing observations are certain, but there is a need to show that mortality rates result from a multiple of causes. In general, it would seem to be a reasonable assumption that health services as such have less influence on mortality rates than general social conditions in economically developed countries.

In view of the difficulty in relating health services to health indices in developed countries, other measures of overall attainment of objectives for a personal health service are sometimes preferable. One of these is the extent to which various income groups have access to the health services. Given the public policy subscribed to by all three countries that there should be equal access to personal health services regardless of income and residence, this level of attainment is easy to measure by appropriate record keeping of use of services or periodic social surveys of the population as to how the health system is being used by the population. There is considerable evidence of this already in the United States and Sweden but only fragmentarily in England.

Concurrent household surveys in the United States and Sweden in 1964 revealed differences. To paraphrase the observations in the research report [9] the results of the income analysis generally supported the postulate that income differences are greater in the United States than in Sweden for physicians' services. Income-class differences were generally found in the United States but not in Sweden for physician services and drugs. Income differences in both countries were small for hospital services and large for dental services. Even though accessibility to hospital services was reasonably thought to be considerably less in the United States than in Sweden, low income on the whole does not at first seem to be a barrier for entry in to the hospital. Since there is much evidence, however, that the poor are actually sicker, it could very well be that "equal" access could result in much more hospital care than at present. Other criteria for comparisons also enter, such as the application of a means test and the "dignity" of the admission process. The findings do suggest that given the present system in the United States, an increase in income or improved health insurance benefits for low-income groups would result in more low-income persons using physician and dental services. Equalizing income differences or introducing dental insurance might also result in greater use of dentists by adults in Sweden where, as of now, adults must pay directly for these services although legislation is pending to make this care free to adults also.

The data on use in England are limited to a study of general practice by Cartwright.[10] Since general practitioners are the sole entry points for patients in England, Cartwright was able to reveal to what extent class differentials exist in how general practitioners are consulted. Since she broke the population into only the middle class and the working class, the categories are rather broad. She reveals that class differentials are

[9] Andersen, Smedby, and Anderson, pp. 86–87.
[10] Cartwright (1967), p. 34.

quite minimal, as one might expect. In fact, the working-class patients appeared slightly more likely to consult physicians than the middle class. There are no data on class for hospital or dental care.

Another objective measure is convenience. It can be assumed that a highly rationalized system can equalize access and depend in part on doing so by the manipulation of queues for various types of services. Queuing is an easy means for a governmental system to allocate scarce resources. Queuing also appears in a nongovernmental system where price is the method of allocation, but the assumption is that an open-market system will increase the supply if queuing is not tolerated.

Systematic data on queuing are singularly lacking in all three countries. The general impression is that waiting lists are common and to be expected in England, particularly for so-called elective surgery. Mechanic, however, argues that these waiting lists are inflated by multiple listings and by people who expedited their care through private practice. The area of elective surgery for which waiting lists are longest is plastic surgery—about eight months (63 percent of total annual discharges, assuming no emergency operations). The second longest waiting list is for tonsillectomy where the queue is six months long.[11] Of course, tied in with the question of queuing for elective surgery is the fact that much less elective surgery is performed in Britain overall.[12] In Sweden there is less talk about queuing. Waiting lists exist but apparently not to the same degree as in England. In the United States the situation is highly variable from area to area. Nevertheless, no country, even one as highly organized as is England, has attempted a rational use of queuing. All three countries feel that there must be some rational means of sorting urgent and nonurgent patients. Still, all three countries take pride in the belief that they are attending to all "urgent" cases.

A final objective criterion, related to the foregoing, is the extent to which a health service protects family financial solvency. This clearly is more of a problem in the United States than in the other countries under consideration. The relatively unpredictable need for health services has been documented extensively. It is unlikely that governmental systems would have arisen if high-cost episodes were not spread so unevenly over families during a given period. With even cost distribution, health services would have occupied the same public policy priority as do minimum food, clothing, and shelter.

[11] Mechanic (1971).
[12] Bunker (1970).

PART FOUR

THE ENDLESS SEARCH FOR THE DREAM

DURING THE LAST 100 years there has been a persistent, albeit uneven, search in the three countries for some sort of distributive justice to mitigate the "slings and arrows of outrageous fortune" embodied in the five contingencies outlined in Chapter 3. But why is there a search for the dream of equality at all? Who cares—other than the deprived and the powerless—whether access to health services is a right? There is hardly a rational answer to this question. The fact that this policy is explicit is a fantastic phenomenon, given the relative scarcity of resources, because it implies that these resources must be shared by some kind of a governmental distributive mechanism. In all three countries no one seriously suggests that the marketplace will distribute health resources equitably for the poor. The most extreme suggestion would have the health services privately owned and operated for profit, with the government buying services for the poor in the same sense it buys food, clothing, and shelter for them. The other extreme is the government's owning everything lock, stock, and barrel—a complete state medical service as in the U.S.S.R. But even England, as represented by the National Health Service, is still far from this type of system although it is felt by many that she is moving in that direction.

Thus the evidence is that the search for the dream is real in its intent; there are differences in methods of attaining the objective. No system, however, can attain equality of access in its pure form. There can only be approximations, but how do we set up criteria of approximations rather than criteria of perfection? Still, the search for the dream continues in all three systems, and these systems reflect their social and political values, including those that are essentially religious in nature. Equality of access to health services is one such value. It is beyond rational debate, but the debate for means to attain the dream is endless.

The dream is embedded in a value called progress. The belief in progress—also beyond debate—emerged in the crucible of circumstances forged by the eighteenth-century rationalists who believed that mankind could harness nature through a particular kind of social and political system that would release latent energy leading to growth in economic productivity and a social surplus for distributive justice. This energy did, in fact, express itself through the industrial revolution. The primary mechanisms are the rational allocation of political power through representative government and the rational allocation of resources through the marketplace. The primary issue becomes the extent to which government intervenes in the market mechanism and the private sector. Orthodox socialism—that is, public ownership of the means of production and distribution—has been applied in varying degrees to the operation of the health services, and such application has been made through the parliamentary process in line with the liberal-democratic traditions established in the nineteenth century.

Thus the Western democracies pride themselves on being able to guarantee individuals both political freedom and an increasing share of the economic surplus. The countries in the orbit of the U.S.S.R. are assumed to have achieved a sharing of the economic surplus by sacrificing political freedom as it is known in pluralistic democracies. In the parliamentary democracies, it is the health and welfare services that have yielded most to the drive for some sort of equalization of consumption of goods and services. The three countries under study present a common core. There are, however, differences between them because of unique national characteristics. The problem of national characteristics is an empirical question: how do we learn about national characteristics and what is a definitive methodology? The methods vary from the notes of a single traveler such as de Tocqueville in America in the early nineteenth century to a social survey of the "civic culture" in the United States and Great Britain by Almond and Verba a few years ago. Both are outstanding; de Tocqueville is almost unbelievable in his foresight. Other observations have been written by good journalists such as Connery on the Scandinavian countries. In trying to relate the development and operation of the health services to the national characteristics of the United States, Sweden, and

England, works of historians, political scientists, sociologists, and anthropologists [1] were drawn upon.

The three countries share a "civic culture" [2] containing both the scientific and the humanistic-traditional culture and enabling these two subcultures to interact and interchange without destroying or polarizing each other. Science and democracy are seen as having a common origin in the humanistic culture of the West. Science is rational, straightforward, and uncompromising in the face of evidence. Civic culture is more difficult to pinpoint in its nuances.

In England, according to Almond and Verba, Britain entered the industrial revolution with a political culture among its elites—the independent aristocrats secure in their local power in the countryside and the emerging nonconformist and self-confident merchants—which was conducive to the assimilation of the gross and rapid changes in the social structure of the eighteenth and nineteenth centuries with containable strain. An amalgam emerged which Almond and Verba called the third culture:

. . . neither traditional nor modern but partaking of both; a pluralistic culture based on communication and persuasion, a culture of consensus and diversity, a culture that permitted change but moderated it. This was the civic culture. With this civic culture already consolidated, the working classes could enter into politics and, in a process of trial and error, find the language in which to couch their demands and the means to make them effective.[3]

The quotation reveals how England was a reference point for the development of parliamentary democracy and the creation of the private and public sectors for both the United States and Sweden. In these countries, however, a major element of importance to the British civic culture

[1] The works listed here as well as those cited throughout the book. United States: Boorstin (1953), De Tocqueville (1956), Galbraith (1958), Ginzberg (1965), Hunter (1959), Lane (1962), Lerner (1957), McConnell (1966), Mills (1956), Monsen (1965), Riesman (1950), Rose (1967), Sutton (1950), Williams (1960). Sweden: Åkerman (1970), Bach (1967), Connery (1966), Dahlstrom (1965), Elvander (1966), Johnson (1963), Myrdal (1966), Rosenthal (1967), Schmidt and Strömholm (1964), Tomasson (1969), Tomasson (1970), Uhr (1966), Zetterberg (1966). England: Almond and Verba (1963), Eckstein (1960), (1962), Gorer (1967), McKenzie and Silver (1968), Nicholson (1967), Orwell (1946), Runciman (1966), Rose (1964), Sampson (1965), Skidelsky (1967), Titmuss (1968), Tuchman (1966), Young (1958), Zweig (1961).
[2] A term attributed to Shils (1961), p. 1.
[3] Almond and Verba (1963), pp. 7–8.

is lacking to this day. England retained, although in an attenuated form, a deference toward government and a class structure supporting it that has been absent in the United States and has disappeared in Sweden. In that sense, the United States since the beginning of Jacksonian democracy in 1829 and Sweden since the abolition of the four statuses in 1862 have been more open systems liberated by the existence of exploitable resources. These were abundant for the United States and reasonably adequate for Sweden. England exploited and controlled both the internal and the empire resources by means of an aggressive and small upper-middle class and an aristocracy. The United States entrepreneurial base became relatively large with a highly mobile labor force. All three became essentially pluralist democracies governed by two major political parties and fluid coalitions of many private interest groups. In this sense the civic cultures of the three countries are similar, but with regard to health services they exhibit a range of implementation.

The United States continues to look at personal health services as a contingency or risk problem for the population. Even in governmental programs, such as Medicare, subsidization of risk is the underlying concept. Ownership of facilities and hiring of personnel, therefore, have low governmental priorities. The risk concept embodies prudent, foresightful, middle-class values and can be successfully carried out in a large affluent consumer society. Furthermore, the social and political ideology seems to support the risk concept. The ideology perpetuates a buyer and seller relationship with funding coming mainly from the private sector. Funding is part of the bargaining and negotiating process in the private sector, and government itself is drawn into this process. The emphasis is on pooling risks rather than "fair shares."

England, on the other hand, seems to prefer a provider-recipient relationship, with funding coming mainly from the public sector. This approach carries on the *noblesse oblige* method of taking care of social problems which now embraces the middle class as well. Health services are part of the very organism of society, and equal access means "fair shares" regardless of whether the economy is expanding or not.

Sweden seems to me to be the least ideological of the three countries as regards methods of implementing the concept of equalizing access. Sweden does not seem to let extreme values, either individualistic or collectivistic, hamper its methodology. Collective, governmental responsibility for individuals in economic difficulty has been a Swedish tradition. Sweden has embodied neither the economic individualization of the United States nor the fair-shares concept of the British. Rather, since 1930 it has very deliberately set out to balance the expansion of the welfare aspects of the state with its ability to pay for them in an expanding economy.

The orientation of each country pervades its debates, discussions, and recommendations concerning the operation of the health services. For 20 years there have been attempts to consolidate public policy both as to objectives and as to methods of organization. In line with these orientations, recent trends are examined.

XI

The Common Ferment Since 1950

Regardless of ownership, sources of funding, and organizations of services, the three countries have been beset by basically the same problems: rapidly rising expenditures due to increasing use and rising prices, perceived shortages of personnel and certain types of facilities, and difficulties in distributing these equitably by residence of the population.

The acceleration of expenditures for health services during the past two decades is causing some consternation. Keeping up with medical technology necessitates a seemingly painful reallocation of resources. Productive and affluent as these economies may be, they still cannot provide everything for everybody. Hence a health service that encroaches on housing, transportation, education, recreation, and a great range of other consumer goods is looked on with mixed feelings.

The public and political concern with rising expenditures did not appear simultaneously in the three countries, indicating different levels of tolerance to costs or perhaps simply ignorance of them. England began to be publicly, hence politically, concerned with rising expenditures in 1949, the very first year after the National Health Service was inaugurated. Expenditure estimates were surprisingly short of actual expenditures that year, £233 million being estimated and £400 million being spent. In fact, as early as 1950 the government established an arbitrary ceiling but, like the American national debt, it had to be lifted. For the first time, England was learning from a simple and single statistic what health services were costing. Having no reference point, the English were shocked. The United States absorbed the increasing expenditures for health services with equanimity until the early 1960s, after which it has become so seriously concerned that it is looking toward universal health insurance as a possible means of slowing expenditures. Sweden, with its much faster pace of increasing cost than either England or the United States, did not become concerned until the late 1960s. The counties and municipalities were then apparently reaching some kind of tax saturation point in order to finance their hospitals.

Now all three countries are converging in their concern for costs, and in all three this concern finds expression in planning, coordination, integration, and regionalization. The long-range objective is the rationalization of the health services to avoid duplication, set up appropriate entry points for patients, structure the range of services so that the right patient is in the right place at the right time (as are the personnel), and avoid "unnecessary" use. After several generations of accumulating importance, the general hospital is to be deemphasized. Furthermore, this is to result in a rational cost structure enabling a clear measure of the relationships among cost, organization, and objectives.

The national attitudes expressed in the tone of the officially sanctioned studies in the three countries reveal crisis mentalities in the United States and England and seemingly calm and slowly paced analyses and reviews of future actions in Sweden before they reach political crisis proportions. As far back as 1952, however, the President's Commission for the Health Needs of the Nation's series of reports were a model of data gathering, hearings from interest groups, and recommendations approaching the Swedish style. Nevertheless, the reports represent an exhausted calmness after almost 15 years of polemics regarding the adoption of voluntary or compulsory health insurance. The relative peacefulness of the Eisenhower era from 1952 to 1960 bore this out. Immediately after, the United States entered into polemics and frantic official studies regarding the aged and scores of meetings where the same data were hashed and rehashed. Never in the history of American health policy had a problem been so thoroughly studied and aired as were the health needs of the aged.[1]

After 1948 England had all it could do to finance and operate the National Health Service, not to mention engaging in studies of it. England's lack of regard for data was epitomized by its having only one statistician assigned to data collection for the operation of a £400 million enterprise. Expenditure data became available, however, with the annual reports from the Treasury, and these were the only data England had, that is,

---

[1] United States Congress, House of Representatives (1961).

the gross expenditure for the Service by components. The policy makers had never seen a magnitude like that for health services before and were astounded by it. The first concern for information, having priority over the operation of the Services itself, was on the remuneration of physicians and dentists, culminating in a Royal Commission on Doctors' and Dentists' Remuneration, 1957 to 1960. This Royal Commission recommended a permanent review body to concern itself with physicians' and dentists' income negotiations.[2] Income negotiations became intense from the very beginning of the National Health Service, and understandably so, because the government was virtually the sole buyer of physicians' and dentists' services. The American concept of "prevailing and reasonable" fees as conceived for Medicare was beyond the comprehension of the Treasury, and, very likely, that of the physicians and dentists as well. It would, of course, have been disastrous in its application.

British health professionals have been accustomed to practicing in much more structured circumstances than either the American or the Swedish, but they are hard bargainers nevertheless. Thus the fact that the problem of remuneration finally reached a Royal Commission level and a permanent review board was set up especially for these professions makes it apparent that the remuneration of the primary professionals is given a high priority. England has a penchant for the concept of "fair compensation," which is defined as compensation fair in relation to other trades and professions as judged by an officially constituted commission instead of as a product of the play of market forces. In a memorandum of dissent, an economist on the Commission, Professor John Jewkes of Oxford University, expressed it as follows: "Such expressions as 'fair compensation' or 'internal relativities' have little value as a guide to policy; and they often lead those who employ them to imagine that they have found a solution when they have only found a phrase." [3]

During the chronic negotiations between the government and the physicians and dentists prior to the Royal Commission Report, there was sufficient concern with the rapidly rising expenditures of the National Health Service from 1949 so that seven years later the problem was submitted to a Committee of Inquiry headed by a Cambridge University economist, Guillebaud. The main concern of the Commission, an evaluation of expenditure trends, was entrusted to Brian Abel-Smith, a young Ph.D. in economics from Cambridge University working with Professor Richard Titmuss of the London School of Economics. Both men were very sympathetic to the concept of the National Health Service and made

[2] Royal Commission on Doctors' and Dentists' Remuneration (1960).
[3] *Ibid.*, p. 159.

as rigorous an analysis of costs as was possible with available data.[4] This was the first overall cost study of the Service. As the main body of data of the report, it deservedly evoked a great deal of attention. Contrary to the assumptions, Abel-Smith and Titmuss showed that from 1949 to 1955 the National Health Service had actually accounted for a decreasing proportion of the gross national product, hence was not the bottomless pit it was purported to be by those who looked only at absolute figures. Furthermore, the authors pointed to the alarmingly low rate of capital investment in the hospital facilities, falling far behind replacement needs, not to mention expansion. Nevertheless, this factual report by no means laid to rest the illusion of an expensive and wasteful service.

In substance, the Committee of Inquiry was a defense of the principle, structure, and operation of the National Health Service. Given the massiveness of the Service and its centralized financing and governing, the Report could hardly do anything else. No health service system is easy to change because after even a few years relationships between the many agencies and personnel reach a level of accommodation that is tolerably workable. As expressed in the Report:

> If fundamental changes were now to be made in the administrative structure, (note: particularly tripartite) new authorities would find themselves faced with new problems and the whole process of adjustment and adaptation would have to be gone through all over again.[5]

Yes, indeed, it would. The Report goes on to say that the framers of the Act did not have

> the advantage of a clean slate; they had to take account of the basic realities of the situation as it had evolved. It is also true that even now, after only seven years of operation, the Service works much better in practice than it looks on paper. That it should be possible to say this is a remarkable tribute to the sense of responsibility and devoted efforts of the vast majority of all those engaged in the Service and also to their determination to make the system work.[6]

The expression "determination to make the system work" recurs in the literature on the National Health Service. It represents a certain commitment to the concept as well as the British capacity to engage in countless negotiating and consulting outside of the formal framework of the Act. This is what the Report must have meant by remarking that the Service

---

[4] Abel-Smith and Titmuss (1956).
[5] Ministry of Health (Department of Health for Scotland) (1956).
[6] *Ibid.*, p. 62.

"works much better in practice than it looks on paper." In seven years the Service had accomplished a staggering task. The population seemed very satisfied and the medical profession, while customarily restive, had made no serious suggestion to tamper much with the Service.

The foregoing evaluation by the Committee was, of course, exceedingly judgmental, but the Report stated emphatically that the current available knowledge of the operation of the National Health Service was inadequate and that there was no factual basis for policy discussions.[7] It was regretted that for the first seven years of the Service the Ministry was without the assistance of a qualified statistician.

Two more quotations reveal the sober hindsight following the euphoria that preceded the inauguration of the National Health Service.

If the test of "adequacy" were that the Service should be able to meet every demand which is justifiable on medical grounds, then the Service is clearly inadequate now, and very considerable additional expenditure (both capital and current) would be required to make it so.[8]

And with regard to reducing morbidity and therefore costs:

There is every reason to hope that the development of the National Health Service will increase the years of healthy life per head of the population, but there is no reason at present to suppose that demands on the Service as a whole will be reduced thereby so as to stabilize (still less reduce) its total cost in terms of finance and the absorption of real resources.[9]

From the inquiry into the National Health Service in 1956 to the late 1960s there was a raft of inquiries and reports into a range of central problems of concern to the Service and to politicians. These inquiries and reports are parallel to ones in the United States and Sweden during the same period, indicating the basic similarities of problems that developed countries face. In England there were inquiries into and reports on the prescribing habits of general practitioners,[10] the supply of general practitioners,[11] nursing staff structure in hospitals,[12] the supply of hospital beds,[13] the role of the general practitioner,[14] hospital medical staffing

[7] *Ibid.*, p. 233.
[8] *Ibid.*, p. 50.
[9] *Ibid.*
[10] Ministry of Health (1959).
[11] Ministry of Health (Department of Health for Scotland) (1959).
[12] *Ibid.* (1966).
[13] National Health Service (1962).
[14] Ministry of Health (1963).

structure,[15] the pharmaceutical industry in relation to the National Health Service,[16] and medical education.[17]

Also investigated were the migration of highly trained professionals other than physicians,[18] a global review of a national plan by the Labour Government in 1965,[19] and a very critical report on the Civil Service.[20] Mention should also be made of the concern with local government as it related to taxing power and relationship to the central government.[21] Finally, two Green Papers (i.e., for public discussion) have been published by the Ministry dealing with recommendations for the restructuring of the National Health Service.[22]

Even the foregoing inquiries and reports do not exhaust the official activities although they certainly reveal the main areas of public concern. In addition there are many private publications dealing with the health services which are alluded to at various points in the book.

All these official inquiries and reports, for my purpose, are of less value for their data—which are hardly abundant in any case—than for the attitudes and policies they reveal of the elements of British life who take an interest in public concerns. The overall impression is one of valiant attempts of a government to handle as gracefully and equitably as possible the complete responsibility for a colossal enterprise—a modern health service. Because of the omnipresence of straitened finances and a heavy commitment to serve the public, the reports are replete with admonitions that physicians be prudent in prescribing services, patients be reasonable in demanding services, and the various authorities work together in a dedicated manner. There is no name calling, no scapegoats, no recriminations—really quite remarkable compared with the American tendency to blame one devil or another. Perhaps the very lack of acceptable alternatives makes the British more accommodating to one another. In the United States options are open, and the very openness of the American health scene makes for vigorous debates and discussions.

Pressures on the National Health Service will, of course, not abate, and this is recognized in the Report of the Royal Commission on Medical Education.

[15] Ministry of Health (Department of Health for Scotland) (1961).
[16] Ministry of Health (1967).
[17] Royal Commission on Medical Education (1968).
[18] Committee on Manpower Resources for Science and Technology (1967).
[19] First Secretary of State and Secretary of State for Economic Affairs (1965).
[20] Committee on the Civil Service (1968).
[21] Ministry of Housing and Local Government (1967).
[22] Department of Health and Social Security (1970).

Advances in medicine are themselves likely to generate greater demands on medical services by making possible the relief or cure of hitherto intractable conditions by extending life expectancy. They are also likely to engender demands for the treatment of conditions, not always trivial, which have in the past been tolerated without much complaint by the general population; this would appear to be reflected in the steadily rising demand for medical care as the economic well-being of society increases. These and other factors tend to complicate the relationship between demand and need and make a precise forecast of either extremely difficult.[23]

Two years later the implicit answer to this statement was the Green Paper in 1970 on the future structure of the National Health Service. The substance of the recommendations was organizational—more money apparently was not considered (because of lack of availability rather than lack of need).[24] Ever since the inception of the Service it has been assumed that the tripartite administrative structure of general and dental practitioners, hospital services, and local public health services was a drag on its efficiency. In the 1970 Green Paper there are strong recommendations to reorganize the Service into 90 administrative jurisdictions embracing all services under each jurisdiction and facilitating the integration of all services under one authority.

UNITED STATES

Various inquiries and reports on the health services in the United States emanate seemingly equally from voluntary and public auspices, revealing a great deal of voluntary citizens' activity. In the public inquiries and reports, representatives of the many interest groups are brought in on the committees, as in England and Sweden. However, once the government appears to be bent on some sort of legislative program—as illustrated by Medicare—the inquiries become "official" rather than "advisory." It seems that the more an inquiry is of an "advisory" character, the more its function is to test the consensus and possibly create consensus. Once such a consensus is established the government can move into more "official" inquiries which are likely to result in legislation.

This process is not as self-conscious as it might appear in retrospect; rather, it seems to be a normal attribute of policy consensus and creation in an interest group democracy. Both England and Sweden reveal the same characteristics, although the process seems more structured and in-

[23] Royal Commission on Medical Education (1968).
[24] Department of Health and Social Security (1970).

stitutionalized than in the United States. It does not seem to occur to private interest groups in these countries to operate outside of the governmental process framework in formulating policy that leads to legislation. They are more likely to work within the framework from the start of an inquiry. There are, of course, voluntary interest groups in England and Sweden that produce data and recommendations touching public policy but appear to be outside of the main stream of the institutionalized political process. Still, the situation in the United States seems to be more open and freewheeling.

In the 1950s and early 1960s the most intense public policy issue on the United States health care scene was medical care for the aged. Concurrently there was a widely and vociferously publicized Congressional investigation into the pharmaceutical industry. The issue was prices and possible monopoly practices and advertising styles.[25] England and Sweden had similar inquiries for similar reasons. The United States hearings were an arena of charges and countercharges, while the British and Swedish inquiries observed the usual decorum of assembling evidence for public policy and information.

Each country was aghast at the increasing expenditures for pharmaceuticals. Still, each country made its peace with the pharmaceutical manufacturers. They had hardly any alternative short of expropriation, and no country was ready for that. Instead, the respective governments became countervailing forces, rather general in the case of the United States, but more specific in England and Sweden by means of price negotiations. Quality standards were essentially a given, hence not controversial.

An example of a governmental stimulus in the United States to gathering data and making recommendations on an important social problem is that begun when Congress passed the Mental Health Study Act in 1955. A series of studies were completed on manpower, social costs of mental illness, and concepts of mental health, culminating in a well-known report in 1961.[26] Although its recommendations were by no means startling—such as deemphasizing institutional care in favor of day care community clinics—the Commission set the tone for subsequent and progressive developments in the mental health field.

The U.S. Public Health Service prepared reports in consultation with relevant interest groups on need for nurses [27] and the problem of area-wide planning for hospitals and related facilities. By 1961 there had been

[25] United States Congress, Senate (1961).
[26] Joint Commission on Mental Health and Illness (1961).
[27] Surgeon General's Consultant Group on Nursing (1963).

sufficient activity in local metropolitan areas toward the creation of hospital planning councils so that the American Hospital Association and Public Health Service participated in a joint report.[28]

Concurrently there was a voluntary group called the National Commission on Community Health Services created by the American Public Health Association (APHA) and the National Health Council (NHC)— APHA being a professional body of public health professionals and NHC being a federation of voluntary health agencies. The Commission was financed by several philanthropic foundations. It was to conduct studies, develop recommendations, and report to the American people. In a highly structured manner the Commission organized its activities under three projects. In one, six task forces were set up dealing with a wide range of problems from environmental health to personal health service delivery systems. In another project there were reviews of 21 "successful" community programs throughout the country. The third project considered communications. The recommendations were quite general and rather self-evident, suggesting the desirability of health service areas, a personal physician for everyone, comprehensive services, effective use of health manpower, and so on. Although there was stress on the voluntary section of the health services, it was suggested that official public health agencies be important vehicles for these recommendations.[29]

The global nature of the recommendations appears to be rather characteristic of the atmosphere of the period. However, subsequent efforts and inquiries reveal more concern with problem specifications and instrumentalities, although underlying them is a great deal of understandable frustration with the intractability and complexity of the problems of increasing use and rising costs. Lacking a strategy, even a general one, such recommendations are therefore put in terms of challenges, exhortations, and moralisms. An exception among the dozen or so reports that were published was one by a political scientist who refreshingly applied some social system–power structure concepts to the analysis of five community programs that were deemed experimental and "successful." His focus was chiefly the feasibility of planning in the American social and political context. He concludes forcefully:

Nowhere in this free-wheeling, pluralistic, local autonomy will planners (health or otherwise) ever achieve the ideal state of affairs in which the unadulterated schemes of technicians become the holy script of political leaders and policy implementors. In any event, sophisticated planners no longer see a comprehensive plan as the end of planning; they now visualize a planning process

[28] Division of Hospital and Medical Facilities (1961).
[29] National Commission on Community Health Services (1966).

in which plans are formulated in broad contexts, offered to policy leaders as guidelines, and subjected to continuing restudy in an interplay between planners and policy leaders.[30]

Nowhere, however, in the report of the Commission is there recognition of the "politics" of health care. The following bland statement is an example of the lowest common denominator characteristic of many Committee reports:

The responsible participation and involvement of all sectors of the community, coordination of efforts, and development of cooperative working arrangements are fundamental to effective action-planning. Health service objectives can be met through processes which provide opportunity for citizens to work together to understand . . . , etc., etc.[31]

In the United States it is difficult to attack a social and health problem comprehensively because of the number and complexity of problems. The approach is more often selective. For example, the government began to show concern about heart disease, cancer, and stroke. These diseases together cause over half of all deaths in the United States. A program for these diseases would be supported by a cross-section of interest groups. Consequently, a noncontroversial legislative proposal was made to improve the care of those suffering from these diseases.

There was a President's Commission set up to look into heart disease, cancer, and stroke, "the highest official recognition that the American Government can give." [32] The legislation flowing directly from this report was passed in 1965, becoming known as the Regional Medical Program dealing mainly with the aforementioned diseases although "related" diseases were included. In the American context this is interesting legislation because it was concerned directly with the prevailing delivery system and how to relate it to the highest level of quality prevailing—that found in the medical schools. It was assumed that some way could be found to coordinate, integrate, and improve the delivery system through government grants as incentives for planning on the local level with medical schools as the main resources for local initiative with no necessary regard for political boundaries. The medical schools needed (and need) money, and this was one way to get them into action.

The Regional Medical Program must appear frightfully messy to British and Swedish observers (and indeed to many Americans who know

[30] Conant (1968).
[31] National Commission on Community Health Services (1968).
[32] President's Commission on Heart Disease, Cancer, and Stroke (1964).

what a rational health system is), but given the federal system and the private ownership of the means of delivering health services, there was little alternative. Even the specifications were general because there was no precedent for them. Guidelines eventually emerged from negotiation and bargaining between the local groups that incorporated themselves for planning purposes and the federal agency thus was given the responsibility of administering the grants. The government had a legislative mandate to do something but did not own anything. All it had was money, a necessary but not sufficient resource.

Glamorous as these diseases were for legislative purposes, the overriding concern continued to be more basic: cost. The President then set up a national advisory committee, which was to deal with manpower but actually ranged over all health services problems, particularly methods of delivery. The Commission membership was composed of the most imposing citizens and professionals the country could produce, and the task forces were staffed by well-qualified investigators. The report reveals the haste with which the Commission had to act, the low level of theoretical and systems thinking in the health field, and its naiveté in suggesting complete reorganization of the health services. It indicates frustration. In neither the public nor the private sector did it find obvious levers, to reshape the health system into the "rational" organization that was sought. Although it suggested an overhaul of the system, the Commission was fearful of giving control over construction of health facilities to areawide planning agencies, because "there is a long history of regulatory agencies becoming defenders of the status quo rather than promoters of innovation and change." [33] Thus the Commission was unwilling to give any agency leverage while at the same time it was dismayed at the prevailing method of negotiation and bargaining between the parties at interest. Alternative models and their consequences were not evaluated; instead the Commission seemed to hope that a "rational" model would be a composite of all advantages with no disadvantages, a systems impossibility.[34]

A year later the government made another attempt at considering the cost of the health services by limiting the scope of the inquiry to hospitals for the obvious reason that they were the largest and fastest-rising cost component in the spectrum of health services. This Committee was created on the administrative level by the Secretary of the Department of Health, Education, and Welfare. Apparently the Secretary was not sanguine about being able to improve the health services immediately. When instructing the Committee he said:

[33] National Advisory Commission on Health Manpower (1967), p. 69.
[34] A detailed critique of this report is to be found in Anderson (1968) (2).

There is not any agreement yet as to what more effective systems of health care ought to look like. . . . Certainly there isn't any agreement as to what the organizing focus of such a better system should be. But it is clear that there is going to be some kind of organizing focus; the system is going to be more inter-dependent than it is now, more interrelated; the various institutions are going to relate to one another in more orderly ways, and this suggests that there is going to be some order.[35]

The American view has been to create some order out of the presumed "nonsystem," which is certainly a "nonsystem" in a bureaucratic and ad-ministrative sense. Nevertheless, the reasons stimulating the investigation in a system that needed more order were the same reasons that led to concern in England, which already had a great deal of order, and later in Sweden, which had some order. The problem of rising hospital cost oc-curred regardless of the system. Again, as in the case of the National Ad-visory Commission on Health Manpower, a distinguished committee was assembled and headed by the dean of a school of business to emphasize the managerial and economic aspects of the hospital industry. To avoid the global pretentions of past reports, both private and public, the com-mittee agreed: "that its specific recommendations would be few in num-ber, high in priority, and pregnant with potential consequences." Recog-nizing a surfeit of recommendations that are really nothing more than statements of desirable goals, the committee also decided that its calls for action must be stated in specific terms, and that they should be capable of implementation in the near and foreseeable future. Finally, it was de-creed that the recommendations must be "doable" rather than conceptual in nature and that they must identify the persons and groups required to act.[36] This was raw pragmatism with a vengeance, but look at the recom-mendations.

The Committee starts with a premise and follows through with princi-ples of implementation, such principles to be capable of particular techniques of management:

Given the extraordinary circumstances resulting from the nature of the health services (need for community and professional "thrusts" rather than the profit motive), the Committee is convinced that the service must remain com-plex and pluralistic, and that its problems are not susceptible of solution either by the introduction of competitive forces or by monolithic centralized planning and controls. No such simplistic solution is sought or proposed in the recom-mendations here, and none is considered feasible.[37]

[35] Secretary's Advisory Committee on Hospital Effectiveness (1968), p. 1.
[36] *Ibid.,* p. 4.
[37] *Ibid.,* p. 10.

The premise puts the Committee in a dilemma, given the Secretary's admonishment to create some order.

Instead, the Committee has considered that the key to solution of the problems of the health service as it exists, with the hospital already established as a central core of medical intelligence and activity, must lie in the introduction of motivation and controls that can be expected to bring shape and a system to a service that has remained formless and disjunctive. The Committee believes an element of planning may be injected into the service in such a way as to compel improvements in effectiveness without directing the application of specific management methods.[38]

The gist of the recommendations is as follows: (1) All facilities should be included in an areawide health service planning agency, and as part of this inclusion the facilities should submit an institutional service plan to the planning agency annually. In turn, the planning agency should publish an areawide plan and guidelines for determining needs and program. (2) The franchising and licensing powers of the state should be used for construction in connection with capital funds from the federal government, which are to be filtered through the local planning councils. (3) Physicians should be brought into the budget planning of the hospitals so that they acquire an understanding of finance. There were recommendations for more detailed internal budget reviews and cost accounting, as well as suggestions for joint purchasing by groups of hospitals and related matters. (4) Finally, it was recommended that health insurance carriers formulate benefit packages that encourage the use of outpatient services rather than hospital inpatient services.

The ideological underpinning for the recommendations is revealed in the following passage:

The Committee is convinced . . . that areawide planning should be done by voluntary nonprofit agencies whose governing boards are composed of leaders of decision-makers representing all elements of the community, including users as well as providers of health services. State authority should be called on only when the areawide planning agency isn't functioning.

A nonfunctioning agency was not defined. The recommendations were a sanctioning and confirmation of trends already established, a legitimate function in itself. They would lead to some degree of "structured pluralism" of the contemporary system, but the extent to which it would bring order of a generally acceptable degree remains to be seen. And this, pre-

[38] *Ibid.*

sumably, is what the American political process is about. "Order" becomes an acceptable balance between contending and cooperating interests. During the same year there was also a national commission on health facilities with the usual array of distinguished experts and citizens called the National Advisory Commission on Health Facilities. Its report went to the President and seemed less concerned with facilities than with their rational organization into regional areas and comprehensive services.[39]

Almost imperceptibly, the Hospital Effectiveness Report flows into the report of the Task Force on Medicaid and Related Programs. This task force seems to pick up the pieces from the fiasco of the Manpower Commission described earlier in that it attempts to think in terms of the financing, administration, and planning of the entire health service system. The latest task force created by the Secretary of Health, Education, and Welfare in July 1969 was charged originally with examining the status of Medicaid, or health services for the poor, a state program that is primarily federally funded. By September the charge was broadened to deal with the entire health service system on the reasonable assumption that health care for the poor was an integral part of health care for the rest of the population, that is, the great majority. Explicitly it was recognized that health care for the poor was a residual, a spillover of health care for the self-supporting. It was now clear that Medicaid had resulted in perpetuating a patchwork of inadequate and underfinanced services among the great majority of the states. Expanding the review of care for the poor to a review of care for everybody had, then, a logical sequence and represents effective political strategy.

Again, this Task Force was made up of the leading authorities in the health field in the United States—from voluntary health insurance, government, all the components of services, and social science. The Chairman heads one of the big buyers of hospital services, the Blue Cross Association. He is no novice in the health field, knowing it well operationally, politically, and financially. Increasingly, the inquiries and reports reveal the participation of social scientists, particularly economists. In this report, particularly, there emerges an idea of basic structural features embodying concepts of competition, incentives, management, and performance criteria.[40]

For the first time there was explicit recognition of the structure and nature of the American social and political system and how a health service system must relate itself to such a society. Although the Task Force

[39] National Advisory Commission on Health Facilities (1969).
[40] Secretary, Department of Health, Education, and Welfare (1970).

claimed it "has no prescription for a new health care delivery system," it came very close to suggesting one, the ideal being group-practice prepayment for the entire population. Although this might be the long-range objective, the short-range strategy was to suggest competition among a variety of delivery systems from which consumers could choose. Presumably the range of types of delivery methods would emerge by quite explicit specifications as to price, range of services, accessibility, and so on to be established by guidelines from the federal government:

. . . to provide all consumers with a greater range of choices among alternative forms of delivery and with the information to make the purchase decision a meaningful one. By thus subjecting the system to increased consumer-purchasing power, responsiveness can be increased without relying solely on centralized planning and direction.[41]

This philosophy was expressed quite humbly. Assuring us that "there are no easy solutions" the concept of competition may well produce greater efficiency in the system:

But competition within the health-care system also has obvious risks. The first risk is that choices made by providers may be guided by self-interest and choices made by consumers may be misguided by ignorance. The second risk is that competition among organizational modes may of itself tend to separate the parts and obscure the view of the system as a whole; one man's pluralism is another man's incoherence.

However, the Report continues:

To safeguard the system against the hazards of provider self-interest, consumer ignorance and fragmentation, it must be managed.[42]

And this managing is to be done by the Department of Health, Education, and Welfare, which reasonably enough is probably the only agency that is supposed to brood over the entire "public interest," given the premise that providers and consumers cannot do it between themselves. In looking after the "public interest," the report actually states a series of unresolvable dilemmas:

As it is envisioned and recommended here, the management function for the health-care system is to be innovative, but not prescriptive; bold, but not authoritarian. It is the intention that the Federal leadership as far as possible

[41] Secretary, Department of Health, Education, and Welfare (1970), p. 5.
[42] *Ibid.,* p. 3.

shall guide, not direct; motivate, not demand; assist, not provide; and evaluate, not ordain. . . .

Somewhere between the extremes of Adam Smith's "invisible hand" and a monolithic governmental health care system is an imposition of logical structure by Government on the health system.[43]

This philosophy surely stems directly from the philosophy of limited government and the economic balancing of the private and public sectors. The ability of any central agency to be as judicious as the quotation implies is something else. Introduction of the competitive model implies inability to set meaningful specifications as to consumer needs and wants and provider performance levels. Hence this report in essence throws the field into the pluralistic model of competition, negotiation, and bargaining while at the same time suggesting that the agency acting in the public interest knows what those specifications should be. The Task Force calls this the "performance-contracting" approach and states that such an approach requires both expertise in contract administration and the ability to define objectives and indicators of performance.[44] In the very next sentence, however, the report reads: "It is generally agreed that the state of the art in measuring the performance of health-care services organization is still relatively primitive." Presumably because of the relative paucity of performance indicators: "The Task Force considers the Health Maintenance Organization [45] concept as an excellent illustration of 'performance contracting' in the health field." This concept is meant to embody a total-package type of health service sold by providers at a contract price for a specified period. The providers then are given the responsibility to police themselves. Given the "primitive" status of performance indicators, the guidelines for performance can be quite general and limited: scope of services, supply, price, and relative ease of access.

In all, there was the supposition that if a good system for claims surveillance and fiscal and utilization control were developed, it would save enough to provide a substantial return on federal investment.[46] This is quite a hope, but could conceivably be carried out by rather arbitrary criteria should such a policy be established. The possibility for saving notwithstanding, the report says that

[43] *Ibid.*, p. 53.

[44] *Ibid.*, p. 60.

[45] The author cannot let the term health maintenance organization pass. It implies that unless services are organized in certain ways "health" is not maintained. It also oversells the degree to which any health service system can "maintain" health.

[46] Secretary, Department of Health, Education, and Welfare (1970), p. 43.

If the Nation is serious about a commitment to a basic floor of health care for all citizens, a considerable expansion of financing and a larger investment of manpower and facilities resources are required. By a simple extension of the $5 billion cost of providing service for 10 million people, for example, one can approximate the cost of providing the same service for 25 million. While this would not be all "new money" and while some economies may certainly be anticipated from the more effective methods of organizing and providing service that have been recommended here, the recommendations for better and more comprehensive service for all who are covered would have a countervailing effect.[47]

As a broadside recommendation the Task Force also suggested more strongly than has been seen up to this time that health agencies should concern themselves with health education of the public. This health education should attempt to change life styles, to reduce cigarette smoking, improve diet so as to reduce heart disease, and change related types of behavior in order to reduce the pressure on the health services. Fundamentally, however, the report is concerned mainly with setting up a "structured pluralism" within which delivery methods compete with each other under governmental guidelines.

SWEDEN

After the universal physicians' service insurance program was inaugurated in 1955, the Swedish government embarked on a series of official inquiries into the same range of problems in the health field as was done in England and the United States. The Swedish reports by comparison are exceptionally good—straightforward, factual, and directed toward limited goals. A remarkable agreement on goals and methods of reaching them make the Swedish reports much less political than the British and American counterparts. The aim is to iron out all major differences between parties at interest regarding particular issues until a majority report can be issued. This takes time. Rarely are there minority reports, a significant exception being tha Höjer report of 1948 recommending a type of state medical service.

The first very fundamental question brought forth after 1955 was that of the regionalization of the hospital services. The counties and the municipalities being more or less self-contained entities for general hospital care, it became apparent that it was not feasible for each county to finance a complete hospital system which would include a major medical

[47] *Ibid.*, p. 13.

center. The government report released in 1958 contained a detailed study of the location of hospital beds and associated specialists throughout Sweden, the distribution of the population, and communication systems. Six alternative plans for regionalization were suggested. A key consideration was the distribution of travel time zones by train, bus, and automobile, and cost of travel. Among the six alternatives there were five to seven major centers designated corresponding to the large urban centers. Eventually, in 1960, an Act of Parliament recommended that the County Councils cooperate in setting up seven hospital regions to provide their populations with the most specialized clinical services at the regional hospitals.

The counties through a federation of county councils, a permanent body, negotiated with the state regarding the details of regionalization. Apparently, these negotiations were conducted with little serious disagreement because the regional plan provided major benefits for all concerned. Even without the large, complex, and expensive central hospitals, the county still had a respectable and basic hospital service under its control. The creation of the county system in 1862 made it almost natural to create regions of counties for hospital services in the early 1960s.

The population of the recommended regions varied from 700,000 to 1,500,000. The central hospitals were planned in connection with medical schools.[48] The Swedes pride themselves on the fact that the counties cooperate voluntarily with the regions. The county that owns and operates the regional hospital has an agreement with the other participating counties guaranteeing a fixed number of beds in the regionalized specialties for each county. The county with the regional hospital is reimbursed by the counties without the hospital on a *per diem* basis. And, incidentally, the state subsidizes these very specialized services—one of the few exceptions where the counties and municipalities do not finance the entire hospital services.

The power of the counties was diminished very little, if at all, by regionalization. In fact, in Swedish opinion the county has been such a successful health service administrative unit that it was given the responsibility for public health officers in 1961 and mental hospitals in 1967 with commensurate taxing power. The former Director-General of the National Board of Health who was in office during the shift to regionalization expressed a typical view of local or county administration:

My experience in a small country has taught me that the responsibility for providing and running health services should be placed with regional and local

48 *Statens Offentliga Utredningar* (**26**, 1958).

authorities, who are living close to the problems and know the needs of the population.

This is followed by a significant conclusion:

It has also been found easier to raise the necessary funds for health purpose at that level.[49]

The British apparently think otherwise and the Americans are trying to find out.

The resolution of the concept of regionalization led to other inquiries fitting naturally into this framework: personnel, particularly physicians, the expansion of hospital and out-of-hospital physicians' services, drug-prescribing patterns, care of the aged, universal dental insurance, mental hospitals, the pharmaceutical industry, and basic problems of taxation, the constitutional and legal basis of local and state relationships, and administration of health and welfare services. These inquiries are summarized in a series of documents bearing on public policy.

The Swedish authorities have been aware for a long time that their country had fewer physicians in relation to population than similarly developed countries. In 1931 there was a study of physician supply which suggested reducing the intake of medical students in order to maintain a reasonably adequate income for physicians.[50] Such reduction was begun in 1935. This viewpoint parallels those found in Britain and the United States. In due course the Swedish medical profession reversed itself, as in the other two countries, and by late 1960s medical students were admitted in greatly expanded numbers. Before long Sweden will have a physician supply approximating that of the United States. A government report revealed that there had been a tremendous expansion in hospital-based physicians between 1940 and 1958, from 1000 to 3000, with no expansion outside of hospitals. Clearly this suggested the policy of increasing the supply of primary physicians also. (It is of interest that Sweden is increasing its physician supply although she has the most favorable health indicators in the world.) The reasons for increasing the physician supply was made explicit in another government inquiry released two years later dealing with the subject of hospital care and out-of-hospital services.[51] The report expresses "an increasing intolerance of shortages

---

[49] Engel (1968), p. 18.
[50] *Statens Offentliga Utredningar* (8, 1961). A general source regarding physician supply in Sweden from 1930 to 1945 is Charney (1969).
[51] *Statens Offentliga Utredningar* (21, 1963).

which despite all advances are found in many instances" [52] and it points to mental health, care of the aged, rehabilitation, certain forms of preventive services, and outpatient services: in short, the full range of the less attractive specialties. Although concerned with rising expenditures, this government report is a sober appraisal of the problem in contrast to the seeming hysteria of the British and American reports. The report states:

> Although we may undoubtedly have a great need for planning which provides some room for expansion of resources outside of the hospital, it is still not likely that a contraction on investment like that of the English would be accepted in our country nor would we recommend anything like that for Sweden. Moreover, we do not have the same institutional structure as England, where health care planning is almost entirely administered by a centralized government. Instead we are striving to keep the decentralization which we already have and which has shown itself capable of building up health services, more and more consistently carried out. [53]

Furthermore,

> Even though the expenditure for health services as a proportion of gross national product must in time spontaneously cease, one must still assume the likelihood that this proportion will continue to increase one or another decennium in the future. [54]

The report counsels that this is the price for a "continuing urgent improvement." It indicates a personnel shortage in hospitals of such intensity that it fears even current personnel will leave because of the work pressure. [55]

The government reports on other subjects mentioned were straightforward, factual, and noncontroversial, even the one on the drug industry. There was concern, of course, with prices, but the negotiations between the domestic drug manufacturers and the government were intense but rational as to cost accounting. [56] There was also thorough examination of drugs as a health insurance benefit, based in large part on a household survey. Even though expenditures for drugs had increased greatly since the inclusion of drugs in 1955, the report discounted the allegations of

---

[52] *Ibid.,* p. 19.
[53] *Statens Offentliga Utredningar* (21, 1963), p. 18.
[54] *Ibid.,* p. 19.
[55] *Ibid.,* p. 104.
[56] *Statens Offentliga Utredningar* (46, 1969).

overuse of drugs. It seemed to accept the current level of use as legitimate.[57]

Other government reports dealt with the aged,[58] dental care insurance,[59] the supply of nurses,[60] mental hospitals,[61] the tax system,[62] local and state relationships, [63] and the administration of social and health services.[64] These are listed to show the depth and breadth of public policy considerations embracing finance, services, and administration. They all fit together in a mosaic of concern for balancing the various interests.

[57] *Statens Offentliga Utredningar* (28, 1960). The household survey was part of a larger survey of the Swedish population conducted in collaboration with a concurrent American survey (Andersen, Smedby, Anderson, 1970). The drug survey was analyzed and published especially for this government report by Björn Smedby.

[58] *Statens Offentliga Utredningar* (5, 1964).

[59] *Statens Offentliga Utredningar* (4, 1965).

[60] *Statens Offentliga Utredningar* (45, 1964).

[61] *Statens Offentliga Utredningar* (50, 1965).

[62] *Statens Offentliga Utredningar* (25, 1964).

[63] *Statens Offentliga Utredningar* (47, 1968).

[64] *Statens Offentliga Utredningar* (49, 1965).

XII

Chronic Problems and Issues

Eᴀᴄʜ ᴄᴏᴜɴᴛʀʏ ʀᴇᴠɪᴇᴡᴇᴅ in this book may be said to have evolved the kind of health service it deserves—no better nor worse than the environing situations allowed. Yet it would appear that in no country is there general satisfaction with the status quo. The belief in progress runs strong, and the very dynamics of medical technology make it impossible to stand still. Each country has evolved a financing and organizational pattern that appears to be congruent with its social and political system. It is not reasonable to expect a country to transcend its own particular social and political system in order to establish whatever may be regarded as a rational model of a health service under which everything else is subsumed. Rather, in terms of resources and organizations, the environing social and political system puts its stamp on the health services.

These observations are hardly novel, but they seem to be ignored in public policy formulation until plans flowing from these policies encounter check points in the social and political system. It may not even be possible to formulate public policy rationally, because of the tremendous number of factors that are involved. Hence each country proceeds according to its own genius, or stupidity, as the case may be.

All three countries have similar operational problems. This indicates, of course, that there are problems inherent in health services administration regardless of ownership control or sources of funds. Each system in substance "works" in that it handles a tremendous volume of patients and

188

carries out a great many technical and complicated procedures. Each system persists in a fashion apparently tolerable enough so that it does not break down although there are prophets of chaos, particularly in the United States and to a degree in England. It requires an amputation of the wrong leg, an inability to recruit nurses, excessive migration of physicians, the ignoring of an emergency call for a heart attack, and rapidly rising costs before the system gets attention. Because every system "works," it permits one to indulge one's bias to a high degree without being called on it.

Problems that are inherent and thus insoluble in any measurable sense must be differentiated from problems that are soluble by some type of conscious act. In the health field it is by no means easy—it seems at the moment impossible—to work out a system that can be predicted to have a net sum of advantages. We do not know how to relate input to outcome in terms of the conventionally desired outcomes such as health indices. There are other indices. Problems in the health services can be classified into operational and equitable. Operational problems are essentially technical and professional, inhering in a particular enterprise. Problems of equity are inherent in a society's values as to who should get what, when, and where, and for how much—in short, a political issue. Political issues come to the fore when a society attempts to implement its concept of equity.

So far, no country or delivery method within it has dared to engage in an experiment to determine what the saturation point of demand for health services might be. Certainly, there is such a point; it is inconceivable that all people would be in physicians' offices or in hospital beds all of the time if the supply were ample. What we do know is that by arbitrary decisions based on quite arbitrary criteria each country sets up controls on demands from the public and from the professional gate keepers, the physicians, well before the theoretical saturation point is reached. These controls can be structural, financial (on the patient or on the entire system), or in terms of an arbitrary limitation of resources according to established standards of equipment and training levels of personnel. England's chief control mechanism is central finance and detailed structure and one entry point for the patient, justified mainly by equity. Almost everyone is looked after by a general practitioner, and the system is financed essentially by a progressive income tax. Sweden's underlying rationale is chiefly one of assuring access and less one of controlling cost because of the decentralized nature of the financing. The United States has no controls to speak of compared to England and Sweden. Although the fee system coupled with insurance that rarely pays full charges may serve as a control on use, use of physicians' services, for example, is greater than that of Sweden and approaches that of England. In effect, the fee system reduces use by low-income groups by making access difficult. The emerging strategy is to establish competing delivery methods, a concept incomprehensible to the British but not to the Swedes. Options exist in the Swedish system as to direct access to a range of physicians: a general practitioner, a specialist, or a hospital polyclinic. Specialists in group practice compete with the polyclinics and at a higher price to the patient. In all three countries the resources and the structures are under pressure from patients and the funding sources are being pressed for more money.

As early as 1954, six years after the inauguration of the National Health Service, a senior administrative Medical Officer of a Regional Hospital Board made a sage observation at the annual conference of the Association of Chief Financial Officers in the Service:

> I think it is impossible to provide an adequate service within existing resources unless a limit is put on the standard of service at the present time. That is a vital statement. We have been through three phases in our expenditure in the health services. To start with we had "money as requested" if you like to put it that way, secondly, "money as required" and thirdly, "not enough money." [1]

This seems to be the refrain everywhere, and no system has worked out a method of determining how much adequacy and equity should cost. Since, in substance, each system seems to work, what is everybody worried about? Fundamentally, there is worry about cost, and philosophically about equality of access. No country seems to feel it has solved the cost problem, but they vary in the extent to which they have solved the access problem of the poor. No country has solved the problem of distributing physicians to areas where they may not like to practice, although the English system has done better at this than the other two countries. The incentives are not good enough and the directing of personnel where to go is not tolerated or if tolerated at all, only temporarily. All systems "work" if the accepted criterion is that all "urgent" cases get attention, a rather elementary criterion and one mentioned often. The common shortcomings are with the refinements of a full-scale health service including services for the acutely ill, the management of chronic illness, preventive services, and rehabilitation. Once a patient is in the system, each system appears to perform well for acute episodes.

No system has been able so far to demonstrate a "proper" health

[1] Association of Chief Financial Officers in the Hospital Service in England and Wales (1955), p. 93.

service system as to quantity of facilities, personnel, and money at a given standard of quality resulting in a given outcome on health indices.[2] At least within the operational ranges of the three countries and developed countries in general, it is misguided public policy to pour more tax money into the systems in order to improve health indices or even to maintain them at their present level. Society might very well obtain a better payoff for health indices by paying attention to other programs such as minimum income, employment, housing, nutrition and life styles and target populations such as infants.

Since general health indices as guides to public policy are not found useful, the indicator of equity is suggested as serving that purpose. Given the pervasiveness of the faith that a modern health service somehow must have some relationship to longevity and better health, it follows that equal access to health services must become a civil right. The equitability of a given health service system appears quite easy to measure with modern data collection methods. From the standpoint of access and quantity of services used, social surveys can reveal how and where selected segments of the population enter the system and with what ailments. Measurements can also be made of those segments of the population who do not use the system.

Another criterion that can be used in systems which have not eliminated charges to patients completely is the extent to which people feel they have difficulty in paying for services out-of-pocket. Still another criterion is the degree to which a system is convenient to use, as measured by length of the queue, waiting time in physicians' offices, and what is entailed in terms of organization and cost to have various degrees of convenience and inconvenience.

This is, at present, not a popular viewpoint. Those who agree with it are cited.[3] The inability to show a relationship between health services

[2] No particular originality for this observation is claimed although I am trying to make it more explicit than have others in relation to public policy; see, for instance, the observation of Thomas McKeown, Professor of Social Medicine, University of Birmingham: "Of the many problems which make the medical task inherently difficult four are outstanding. They are: uncertainty about objectives; lack of indices of achievement; difficulty of assessing priorities within the wide range of measures on which health depends; and the costliness of procedures relevant to health." McKeown (1966), p. 10.

[3] John Fry, a British general practitioner, wrote: "As for qualitative indices, it is doubtful whether the *form* [italics added] has made any ultimate difference to the health of Soviet, American or British citizens." Fry (1969), p. 231.

A team of American, Swedish, and British medical researchers concluded: "Present information does not suffice to permit a judgment as to whether we and health indices leaves physicians interested in health services organization understandably frustrated, given their concept of outcome. Because of their orientation social scientists feel congenial with other indices of outcome such as degree of access, convenience, and satisfaction although there is not necessarily agreement as to how the services should be financed and organized. An American sociologist, for example, reviewed the scattered studies of use of services in England by social class and came to the conclusion that the lowest social class makes the greatest use of physician and in-hospital services. He then takes the view that the National Health Service is equitable, although he did not attempt to make a judgment about its adequacy. He recognized that there might be a major conflict between equity and adequacy, and the challenge in the future may well be how to advance adequacy without jeopardizing equity.[4] This is, indeed, a generic problem in all countries that purport to strive for equal access. Eli Ginzberg, an economist, seeing no relationship between health expenditures and general health indices, suggests limited governmental expenditure. Assurance and convenience, he agrees, should be brought in the private sector.[5]

A British economist and a severe critic of the National Health Service concept argues that it is fallacious to suppose that health services have a great investment potential. They should be treated as a general-run consumption good. Expenditures for health services may be high or low according to this view, but at least there need not be an expectation of future dividends either in increased production or diminished illness.[6] In this concept the state remains responsible for the poor but should buy services from the private sector. A senior economist and his wife from Oxford University observed that the National Health Service actually neglected the long-range payoffs that might be possible, such as improvement of facilities, medical research, and specific preventive measures.[7]

are prodigal with our resources (as measured by health indices) or whether our provisions for care are appropriate or even insufficient." Peterson et al. (1967), p. 776.

Former Surgeon General of the United States, William Stewart, and Philip E. Enterline concluded: "There is no clear evidence that the increases in physician utilization apparently resulting from the N.H.S. improved the health of the adult population." They suggest that N.H.S. had a possible effect on the infant mortality rate, and they were quite certain that there was an increase in use among lower-income groups and groups not previously covered." Stewart and Enterline (1961).

[4] Rein (1969), p. 810.
[5] Ginzberg (1970).
[6] Lees (1961), p. 29.
[7] Jewkes (1963), p. viii.

Each country continues to work out its health services by trying to be responsive to the various parties at interest with open discussions, debate, political power plays, and perhaps even some information for policy purposes.

This is hardly to say that the parties at interest in the health field are negotiating and bargaining as equals. Perhaps equal bargaining positions are neither possible nor necessary. In a professional service we must rely on the health professional to set standards of training and performance, which in turn results in a certain volume and cost of services. At many points the professionals should be and are challenged as to whether they must have certain equipment and arrangements simply because they want them. In each system the professional is given the final decision about the level of training and performance and, so far, the layman— patients or politicians—have in the last analysis deferred to the professionals' judgment. The acceptance of professional judgment has been generous in the United States and Sweden [8] and grudging in England— enough to keep the physicians at their posts, even though there is alarm at the rate of emigration and sporadic threats to strike.

It would appear that England has the happiest public and the unhappiest professionals of the three countries. It would also appear that the United States has the happiest profession—although feeling besieged —and the unhappiest public. Sweden might have been said to have the happiest physicians and possibly also the happiest public, but the profession is beginning to feel pressed in the face of the results of the negotiations regarding salary and working condition for hospital-based physicians. Although it would seem that the American public is least happy, it is doubtful if the broad middle class is willing to give up the options, convenience, and quality, which a highly structure service is not likely to give.

There is pressure on each system to coordinate, integrate, and plan. It is felt that somewhere there must be a holy grail not yet discovered which will reveal the main features of a rational system. This feeling is pervasive even in England, which has the most logically structured system of all three countries. And England hopes to go one final step fur-

[8] In a Swedish study of budget decision making in the hospitals there is a series of quotations from finance committee chairmen of the county councils whose chief official concern is the financing of the hospitals and advising the County Councils. They reveal that the Swedes until now, at least, have worked within generous cost limits: "We have been in the economic situation that we have not had to be prudent. Here they (the physicians) get what they want" (p. 97). "When a physician says that something is necessary for health care, one has to have an icy stomach to say no, particularly if they say that they cannot take responsibility for the service otherwise" (p. 147).

ther in this coordination by abolishing the tripartite structure, thus clearing the obstacles to the integration of the general practitioner, the hospital, and the public health services. The medical profession retains great influence, however. Eckstein, for example, has written convincingly about the close working relationships between the British Medical Association and the Ministry of Health. He reasons that the "collectivization" of medicine, as he puts it, has led to the growing corporatorization of the medical profession resulting, de facto, in giving the B.M.A. great powers. He observes that this is simply a natural outgrowth of the "corporativism" of British society, making pressure group politics easier because of the great web of interconnections. Eckstein elaborates:

In its present form (the BMA) is a vast, highly bureaucratized and wealthy organization; it is the creature rather than the victim of public medical policies; and, far from being involved in constant warfare with the Ministry, it is engaged in constant cooperation with it—a highly useful adjunct to the Ministry's machinery of administration which, had it not already existed, the Ministry would have had to invent.[9]

This is quite an observation, given the current trends in all three countries of attempting to bring physicians into hospital financial and budgeting discussions and decisions.[10]

Perhaps it may well be better to deal with the medical profession simply as another interest group pushing on the scarce resources for their individual patients rather than encouraging them to think institutionally and administratively. As a Swedish clinical department head has said, "A department head who does not carry through what he regards as desirable does not look after his job." The job of the administrative staff is to look after the resources in terms of the community; the job of the physician is to press on the resources in favor of the patient. Although this strategy does not appear to be congenial in the British context, it should certainly be congenial in the American context, if the United States intends to take the concept of "structure pluralism" seriously. It seems that the Swedes have some respect for this concept both in principle and in

[9] Eckstein (1960), p. 48.
[10] A director of one of the Swedish counties, for example, evoked interest in the Swedish medical journal who suggested that in the interest of "rationalizing" the Swedish health service the physicians need to enter into planning and economics. He feels that the hospital could be run more like a business and in the next breath he throws in the warning that "by so doing does not mean that the humanitarian, the so-called personal care, cannot be taken into account." This view appears as an inherent conflict everywhere. Lindencrona (1966).

practice, given their pervasive belief in interest group pluralism. Elvander describes this characteristic in his study of Swedish interest group politics.[11]

As is obvious, the American political scene is hardly tidy, given the diversity of American political interests—ethnic, religious, and sectional—none of which Sweden needs to contend with.[12] Sweden's homogeneity is, therefore, much less challenging to the health services operation than America's heterogeneity.

Professional freedom, that is, the prerogative of the physician to diagnose and treat as he sees fit within the system, is respected. The British and Swedish medical professions rarely, if ever, complain about this important aspect of a government medical service. The American profession continues, of course, to be fearful. What physicians in all three countries watch carefully, however, is the method and amount of payment. Powell, a former minister of Health, observed:

> . . . the unnerving discovery every Minister of Health makes at or near the outset of his term of office is that the only subject he is ever destined to discuss with the medical profession is money . . . cynically, but unjustly, he may be tempted to assume that this is because money is the only thing the medical profession cares about. It is not so; what has happened is that the nationalized service makes money the sole terminology of intercourse between profession and government.[13]

He might have added: "or any third payer."

Proper practice conditions, such as equipment, facilities and supporting personnel, and patient load, are a given and are lived with, but remuneration is a chronic issue. On a worldwide canvas, for example, Glaser observes after reviewing remuneration methods in 16 countries: "The payment of doctors is an impassioned issue throughout the world." [14] He begins his book with the sensible assumption that "Profes-

---

[11] Elvander (1966).

[12] In this connection it is amusing for an American to observe the Swedish government's great concern with the few thousand gypsies and the Lapps in the North. Both of these minority groups have life styles very different from the usual Swedish society. The Lapps stay in the North, however, and benefit a great deal from the Swedish welfare state measures. The gypsies continue to be nomadic over the entire country and are an annoyance to the smooth operation of a rational welfare state. There are also accounts from England of the difficulties of assimilating immigrants from Asia and the West Indies with different life styles.

[13] Powell (1966), p. 14.

[14] Glaser (1970), p. 3.

sional institutions and their incentive systems . . . are supposed to make possible rather than obstruct the realization of the profession's mission." [15] He comes to a conclusion dismal for current planning: "No system has devised payment formulae or administrative procedures that strike the perfect balance." [16] A continuing tension , is, therefore, inherent between payment methods and desired results regarding quantity, quality, and accepted costs.

The ideal payment method from the point of view of the planner is salary; the persisting ideal of the physician is fee-for-service. Indeed, it can be observed that any other method of payment than fee-for-service is tolerated by the medical profession only as long as the physician is permitted a degree of private practice or a high income, or both. As long as the private sector of a mixed economy is the reference point for income levels and the safety valve for physicians for extra income, government can more easily negotiate a salaried service successfully by allowing options. In England, the hospital consultants were permitted to have a private practice in addition to their consultant posts (not to mention the added income from Merit Awards). In practice 70 percent of the consultants work in the hospitals part time and carry on a private practice.[17] The remaining 30 percent are usually the specialists who require a full-time hospital base such as radiologists and pathologists.

The general practitioners are permitted to engage in private practice, and a majority of them do so to various degrees. A very small percentage, at most between 2 and 3 percent, are engaged purely in private practice.[18] There may be some question about the future of private practice

[15] *Ibid.*, p. 1.

[16] *Ibid.*, p. 296.

[17] A British journalist counted 850 physicians in 150 houses in Harley Street, London. There are additional ones in Wimpole Street. In an informative review of private practice he said: "Harley Street wouldn't flourish if its comforts weren't worth purchasing. There's no reason why the comforts should not be handed out in private consulting rooms attached to hospitals, with all the equipment and facilities to hand, and this is likely to happen. But not just yet." Ferris (1965), p. 43.

[18] This estimate is Mencher's (1970), based on estimates done primarily in the 1950s, since little new information was available. Cartwright (1967) p. 275 has the only new information, which is based on a social survey of patients, *not* physicians. She found that although less than 1 percent of her respondents went only to a private doctor, 4 percent of nonrespondents for whom this information could be obtained went only to a private doctor. Adjusting for all nonrespondents, users of private doctors in England range from a minimum of 1.2 percent of the population to a maximum of 4.7 percent, the latter being con-

in England, but currently it certainly exists.

One of the difficulties in sustaining private practice, however, is the division between general practitioners and specialists, resulting in a dual voluntary insurance system. The voluntary plans such as the British United Provident Associations have usually written insurance for specialist services only, that is, N.H.S. consultants, who admit their patients to the approximately 2500 private beds (2.5 percent of all general beds) or to the slowly increasing number of nonprofit private hospital beds sponsored by the Nuffield Provincial Hospitals Trust and others for this thin layer of private demand. The British Medical Association has also sponsored medical insurance for general practitioners but with hardly spectacular results, only about 600 general practitioners out of 20,000 having signed up. The general practitioners were supposed to contribute $25 each for a capital fund to reach over $500,000, but the contributions fell drastically short.[19] The British general practitioners appear to be very nonentrepreneurial, as compared to their American and Swedish counterparts. This may also be true of the specialists. British specialists play it rather safe by expanding from a stable consultant position in the hospitals to private practice and insurance.

In Sweden hospital-based specialists were accorded options to earn extra fees in the polyclinics attached to the hospitals and from patients who sought them on an outpatient basis privately. For private patients the specialist paid the hospital a symbolic sum of 5 Swedish crowns ($1.00) for each patient. The physicians practicing outside of the hospital (except the public health officers) did not enter into a contract with the government through its sickness insurance funds, hence had no negotiated fee schedule. Furthermore, the patient pays the physician directly and is reimbursed by the sickness insurance fund on submission of a claim.

The patient also pays part of the polyclinic charge. It is regarded as a sensible means to make the patient think about money, even if minimally, before a physician's service is sought. In the British context a fee at point of service, however small, is beyond serious consideration. One third of the Swedish physicians in practice outside of the hospital, hence with no hospital appointments, are certified specialists.[20] They prefer to

sidered extremely unlikely. Since physicians in private practice will have a smaller number of patients than NHS physicians, Cartwright's study bears out Mencher's estimate quite well.

[19] Jones (1967).

[20] *Statens Offentliga Utredningar* (8, 1961), Om Läkarbehovoch Läkartillgång, p. 161.

develop their earning power outside of the hospital hierarchy and not wait for the slow pace of promotion. In recent years these specialists, under the aegis of a corporation sponsored by the Swedish Medical Association, have been establishing specialist medical groups in the larger cities. As of 1968 there were 17 group practices and 174 full-time specialists in the groups.[21]

The professional and entrepreneurial attitudes do not mix in England. It has been difficult, for instance, to induce general practitioners to set up group practices until the last few years. In part, this has been due to the capitation method of payment, in which the general practitioner has to finance his entire practice from the capitation. The Local Health Authorities were to be the chief source of capital funds for health centers, but they rarely seemed to have any money. The government now has a loan system to assist general practitioners in capital financing of group practice facilities and also provide a small investive payment. In England group practice is conceived of as a group of general practitioners who share the workload and stand by for one another. Referrals are made to the hospitals when specialist services are deemed necessary.[22] The general practitioner concept has strong official support in England.

In the United States private group practices have been increasing for many years and exhibiting a great diversity.[23] The open health system and the entrepreneurial attitudes of American physicians facilitate this movement, but there is still worry over the concept of the primary physician. A partial American answer has been to make general practice a specialty.

The physicians in Swedish group practice are on salaries, and the group collects fees from the patients in the same way as the general practitioners. It was Rosenfeld's observation that the Swedish Medical Association is sponsoring this movement, quoting one S.M.A. official, "because it wants to strengthen the private sector and it wants a place to work if there is a strike or a lockout in Sweden. In that case these groups

[21] Rosenfeld (1969).

[22] There are now 229 health centers in England and Wales, a great increase since 1968 when there were 93. Still, only 6.5 percent of the general practitioners are involved. Working partnerships are another matter. Less than one fourth of the general practitioners are now in solo practice. Curwen and Brookes (1969), p. 945.

[23] There are now over 6000 groups involving 40,000 physicians or 13 percent of physicians in practice. The number of physicians per group ranged from 3 (the minimum necessary to be defined as a group) to 850, and methods of payment varied widely. McNamara and Todd (1970).

could be centers in which doctors could work and give medical service outside the hospital. It is a protection for all doctors." [24] It also, of course, gives patients options for appointments at the polyclinics for a higher price.

A bone of contention since 1955 has been the privilege of the hospital-based physician to earn extra fees in the polyclinics and from private patients in his own quarters. Given the fee arrangement, the radiologists and laboratory-based physicians in many instances earned enormous incomes over and above the $14,000 base salary they had from the hospital services. There were reports of incomes as high as $75,000 to $100,000 a year. As is normally the case in a fee system, there is an enormous range in earning ability among specialists. The government began in early 1969 to negotiate with the hospital-based medical profession to abolish the fee system altogether and put everyone on a full-time salary according to grade, ignoring specialty differences. Accounts have it that the negotiations were exceedinly intense.[25] In fact the physicians were very close to a strike as the customary Swedish matter-of-factness evaporated.

In view of the fact that a full-time salary was sought by the government, length of the working week then also came into question, as well as the expectation by the hospital administration that the physicians be at a certain place at a certain time. Furthermore, were physicians to be paid for the time they were on call but not at the hospital?

The final agreement involving hospital-based physicians and public health officers seems generous, indicating the bargaining power of the profession when it is organized. The professors received the highest settlement, about $30,000 (more than the Director-General of Health and Welfare) with categories down to the lowest at around $12,000. Of the 7000 physicians, 1700 emerged with reduced incomes and the rest with increased or the same incomes. The cost to the counties and the State remained the same, but the distribution among the physicians was changed. Furthermore, $8 million was set aside as a pool for three years for physicians whose incomes were to be reduced in order to lessen the impact. The fee system has thus been eliminated for hospital-based physicians and health officers. The patient now pays $1.40 for each polyclinic visit to the hospital rather than to the physician, and the hospital collects

[24] Rosenfeld (1969), p. 68.
[25] These are not exhaustive but are sufficient documentation for the purpose. From *Svenska Läkartidningen*, **66**, 662, 1202–1207, 2123–2132, 4625–4628 (1969), **66**, 923–930 (1970). A summary appeared in *Dagens Nyheter* (1970). As can be imagined, the newspaper publicity was extensive and controversial.

the remainder from the sickness-insurance fund. The general practitioners and specialists outside of the hospital are now wondering if they are
next.

The medical professions in all three countries continue to wonder what
is going to happen depending on the particular stage of evolution in
each country. In England the general practitioners would react to going
from capitation to salary; in Sweden they would resist going from fee-for-
service to capitation. In the United States there is resistance to any attempt to regulate fee-for-service. United States physicians are as unpre-
pared for a systematic counterstrategy as were the British and Swedish
professions.[26]

Some of the leadership in the British medical profession and a few
economists are continuing to hope for a viable private medical sector
which can be a counterweight to the National Health Service rather
than, as currently, a safety valve.[27]

A few of the economists associated with the Institute as advisors were
commissioned by the British Medical Association to examine the financing of health services and reporting in 1970.[28] Seldon was one of the
economists commissioned by the B.M.A. and in an earlier publication he
did not appear too sanguine about changing the N.H.S.: "After 20 years
the roots of the NHS may now be so deep that they require an instrument as pointed and penetrating as the voucher to dig them up and re-
plant them." [29] The very thought of changing the N.H.S. in any substantial degree raises as strong feelings among its proponents as those of

---

[26] I have entertained the uncharitable notion that if more women were brought
into the health services as primary care custodians as in Eastern countries, it
might be possible to cut costs and have a more tractable profession than has
been true of the West with its almost exclusively male composition. Eastern Europe and U.S.S.R. have a very large female component in its medical corps,
concentrated largely in the primary care sector of the delivery system.

[27] This idea finds expression largely through the publications of the Institute of
Economic Affairs founded in 1957 as an educational trust, a conservative coun-
terpart to the venerable Fabian Society. The least this institute has done—no
mean feat in the British context—was to bring some serious attention to the
very concept of the National Health Service: comprehensive care free at time of
service and supported from general taxes. The Institute does not limit its attention to the health field but explores other economic problems in Britain. The
first of the series on the health service was by Lees, already cited. The other research monographs related to the health service are by Seldon. [Seldon and Gray
(1967), Seldon (1967).]

[28] Jones (1970).

[29] Seldon (1968).

opponents to universal health insurance in the United States in the forties. The question is almost beyond rational study and discussion, and becomes enmeshed in the concept of equity. This concept naturally cuts across all health and welfare considerations because it is essentially an income-distributive mechanism. The opponents of universalism, that is, services the same and free for all, believe that if health services were open to purchase as desired through both compulsory and voluntary insurance and a public subsidy were provided for the care of the poor, there would be a net larger supply of funds for health services than in the current centralized funding of the National Health Service. Moreover, the poor could be made a prime target so that special problems that may be obscured in a universal health service can be systematically alleviated. Indeed, proponents of universalism such as Titmuss, Abel-Smith, and Townsend [30] do point out the inequities in current universalism because of deficient attention to special problems among the aged, widowed, and handicapped, many of whom are poor.

[30] Abel-Smith (1967), Titmuss (1968), Townsend (1968).

XIII

Postscript and Prognosis

IT DOES NOT REQUIRE BOLDNESS to predict that in all three countries the drive toward increasing coordination, integration, and planning will continue. The concept of planning itself needs critical examination. Its successful application does not necessarily depend on the level of skills and sophistication. The problem is: do we know what we are doing when we plan in relation to resources, structures, and goals? My reluctant skepticism toward rational planning and structuring of services lies in our inability to set up specifications with any degree of precision; hence I tend toward "loose" systems. England never thought she could afford such a system even if she were able to conceive of one; Sweden has been doing so for a long time. In the United States a "loose" system is congenial, but now it may be regarded as too wasteful. England continues to want one gatekeeper—the general practitioner or a health center—and one central source of funds. Sweden wants a specified range of gatekeepers and several sources of funds. The United States seems to be moving to the Swedish pattern, one that Sweden arrived at intuitively: diversity of funds and options in entering the system.

The problem of the kind of gatekeeper remains a thorny one: England wants a general practitioner, pure and simple, but this is a concept that flies in the face of professional desire to specialize and have high status. It would seem to be a truism that status cannot be decreed no matter how many public utterances of appreciation and need are made. Perhaps specialization has reached the end of the road, and now medical students are wishing to become generalists—an unlikely prognosis. The British are more anxious to perpetuate the general practitioner pattern than either the United States or Sweden, as expressed in official studies and pronouncements from both the B.M.A. and the Ministry.[1] The Swedes control the specialist appointments in the hospitals, but permit physicians without hospital appointments to specialize or be general practitioners as they please. The development in the United States appears to be spontaneous depending on the individual physician's desire and capacity to determine his own practice style within a wide range of alternatives and combinations of alternatives compared with Sweden and England. Conceivably, this very freedom can lead to supermarket impersonality as American physicians in private practice enter more and more into private group practice units to spare themselves from immediate and direct access from patients, as well as enabling better standby services at night and on weekends. The British general practitioner, so far, is directly accessible to his patients, although in large cities this is also a problem now for emergency services.

Authorities in all three countries expect that costs are going to increase into the indefinite future. My view is that a diffusion of sources of funds will result in a net increase in money beyond that yielded by a single source of funds, because of lack of control over one source. There is room for debate on this point as, for example, Chester's asserting that the amount of funds is largely a function of the status of the British economy when the government faces many competing claims for high priority in the allocation of economic resources.[2] The tradition of British government, like the American government, has not been noted for its generosity in financing health and welfare programs, and a health service requires a relatively tremendous outlay. The Swedes have proved to be relatively generous, but then Sweden has not been dominated philosophically by the Manchester liberals. The tradition of niggardly financing of public health and welfare programs is difficult to overcome in both England and the United States. Even a Labour government is reluctant to tax heavily. It has to stay in power, and as Marquand, a labour M.P. observed, this is the dilemma of democratic socialism: the gap between poor minorities and the rest of society.

. . . cannot be closed merely by soaking the rich, however desirable soaking the rich might be on other grounds. It can only be closed by a deliberate redistribution of income, away from the comfortable and toward the poor. In a de-

---

[1] See British Medical Association (1930), Godber (1969).
[2] Chester (1968).

mocracy, this can only be done if the majority—or at least a significant part of the majority—agree. And the moral of the last five years of British history (1964–1969) is that the majority are not going to agree unless the overall rate of growth is high enough for their own living standards to improve in absolute terms while the redistribution is carried out.[3]

Abel-Smith and Townsend, however, believe that the gap between private affluence and public squalor can be closed without any economic growth.[4] Politicians like Marquand and Crossman, the latter former Minister of the Department of Health and Social Security, feel that this view is unrealistic and that the gap cannot be corrected without a fairly rapid rate of economic growth.[5]

Both Swedish and American politicians are clearly of the opinion that redistribution needs to be accompanied politically by an increasing gross national product. The Swedish welfare state is founded on this concept. "Fair shares" are easier to attain when there is continuously more to share. Sweden has had the advantage not only of rapid economic growth but of being a small homogeneous country with much narrower extremes of both income and social class than the United States or England, but also no economic disruption by war. This undoubtedly accounts in large part for the success of the Swedish health care system, a system that would reveal many serious defects if it were subjected to the deep stresses and strains of the American and British systems.

The prognosis that health services will continue to require more money is also an easy one to make. None of the three countries feel they are doing enough for prevention, long-term illnesses, or rehabilitation. In view of the resources required by elaborate procedures such as open-heart surgery, dialysis, and organ transplants, these procedures will drain off resources needed for the less spectacular services. It may also be that money will not buy the humane services required for the dull, uninteresting, and unrewarding patients with long-term chronic illnesses. It will likely be possible to recruit for the highly skilled tasks—physicians and technicians—but not for the less technically skilled caring tasks. More reliance will need to be placed on relatives. It may be that surgery will be so successful that procedures associated with it will require a very substantial portion of the gross national product simply to forestall death for a few more years unless society is able to face horrendous decisions and decide to forego open-heart surgery in favor of humane long-term care,

[3] Marquand (1969), p. 490.
[4] Abel-Smith (1966).
[5] Crossman (1967).

for example. This may be the subconscious reason why rising costs are viewed with so much alarm. Allocations of priorities will be distressing, to say the least.

It is predictable that policy makers in all three countries will be looking for more information—cost per case, utilization rates by geographic areas, personnel-population ratios—but unless sophisticated systems analyses are improved, it makes little difference whether the Liverpool area has a higher or lower surgical rate than a county in Sweden. The tendency is to adopt the lowest rate of something because it costs less and there is no evidence that reducing use or facilities or personnel does any harm to the population as measured by mortality and morbidity rates. If we could go one step further and explore social-psychological variables such as assurance and satisfaction and variables measuring equity, we would have an objective measure for public policy formulation. The application of these measures does not appear to be immediate, however.

This survey of three countries has been sobering because little has been learned about what constitutes an adequate health service unless one relies mainly on the concept of equal access as a measure of adequacy. Still, it is certain that some "good" is being done. The public obviously wants health services; otherwise politicians would not enshrine access to health services as a civil right. Current methodology is not good enough to determine the elements and operation of an "efficient" system—cold comfort to policy makers who wish to make judicious decisions involving a visible portion of the gross national product. Even in a political bargaining context, systematic information is necessary in order to provide more intelligent bargaining, as stated by the former chief of the Bureau of the Budget of the United States government, Charles L. Schultze. A tidy and self-contained program may be suggested, supported by reams of facts, but

. . . All too often public programs in such fields as education, health, crime control, urban development and pollution control ignore the system of incentives and structural relations within which social policies must operate. A plan and a fistful of money will not be enough to achieve the objectives of public programs if the plan runs counter to the motivations, rewards, and penalties of the public and private institutions which must carry it out.[6]

Maybe this is why all three health systems reviewed in this book "work." Lacking systematic specifications, the politicians and other interest groups are responsive enough to the different pressures so that each

[6] Schultze (1969), p. 5.

system operates in a tolerable equilibrium. But this equilibrium can be upset at any moment as a new pressure group emerges, a technological breakthrough is made, or more refined concepts of distributive justice are adopted by the body politic. It is currently least stable in the United States, because this country has no global national health insurance program. A relatively stable equilibrium is sought by means of a government health insurance program because there are then no global alternatives left and a country hopes to settle down with the framework of organization and funding at which it finally arrives. Still, in the United States a national health insurance program will hardly settle the issues of cost, volume, quality, and access. The private sector will bulge out any time that government policy seems unduly restrictive to a large segment of the relatively affluent American public. The logical consequence then is, of course, a continuation and institutionalization of two grades or levels of service, one for the low-income who cannot afford to buy outside of the system and one for the comfortable.

The United States stands at the threshold of long-range shifts in methods of delivering and financing services as revealed by the many legislative proposals now being put forth. These proposals range from a structuring of the health services on the British model to one limiting government provisions to the poor and the aged. The application of the British model is exceedingly unlikely, if not unthinkable in the American context. There are too many church-owned hospitals for one thing, and it is unlikely that American legislation will limit entry to the system solely through a primary physician such as a general practitioner. What will emerge from this ferment is likely to be a form of structured pluralism with various sources of funding mainly under government aegis, and various types of complementary and even competing delivery systems, resulting in options on the part of the public. Special provisions will likely be made for the poor so that they can participate more equitably in the mainstream of American medicine depending on level of funding. The controversies regarding group practice, group practice plus prepayment, and methods of paying physicians and institutions will be in a constant ferment and development. Directives toward certain types of structures of services and their coordination will be minimal; rather, inducements to change will be by financial incentives to or minimal control on providers.

This approach is necessarily expensive compared to the British system of a tightly controlled single source of funds funneled through a single type of structure, tied to an economy requiring constraint on expenditures for all purposes. The Swedish system has turned out to be expensive because of a loose sense of expansion and no central control over funding. All three systems, however, face the same pressures of people and technology, and the seductive suggestion that the presumed efficiency of the industrial production line be applied to the delivery of medical care is viewed as a solution. Thus there will be greater attempts at some form of rational budgeting in relation to objectives, needs, and demands, and some form of, at least, short-range incremental planning, such as five-year plans revised every year.

But let us be forewarned about this: a health services system can never approximate the industrial model for rationality as long as patient perceptions and needs are as varied as they are and the physician is accorded the professional freedom to diagnose and treat as he deems necessary. These two factors will continue to be sufficiently indeterminate to preclude tidy and rational models of health service organization which can be set up by scientific yardsticks as to proper finance, proper use, and proper organization. All countries will continually feel their way into the ever-emerging medical technology as best as they can and will continue to be worried about the cost of coping with medical casualties in relation to other desires for goods and services.

The foregoing is in contrast to the usually glowing predictions of some sort of medical care utopia where everyone will have equal access to services and where there will be a proper balance of curative, preventive, and caring services. The latter means compassionate management of long-term and intractable illnesses which virtually all of us will experience as we age. It does not seem reasonable to hope that cure and prevention can become so effective as to eliminate long-term disabilities. Society has to arrive at a point soon—and already there is increasing interest in dignified death and dying—where we must plumb the depths of our basic values and question the concept of continuing life as an end in itself. It is difficult to justify heart transplants because of the potential sense of state of emergency the social system must continue to absorb as a recipient waits for an accident to happen to a donor, for example. The construction of a mechanical heart will not alter the basic problem of the heroic efforts to prolong life. These observations flow, of course, from deep value judgments, but they do have implications for how we structure, finance, and deliver health services and how we allocate our resources in relation to both our overall needs and desires and priorities within health needs themselves.

Research and critical observations have compelled the drawing of one reluctant conclusion after another. The possibilities for completely rational planning, adequate measurements of efficiency of operation and cost, adequate measure of effectiveness by use of the usual health indices, incentive systems strong enough to induce health professionals to move to understaffed areas, and so on seem beyond reach for a long time to come.

All three health systems moving into greater organization and bureaucratization in order to control cost against the vast reservoir of real or imagined ills (in health services administration both are real in their consequences). This move will be rationalized by claims to spurious efficiency. There will likely be increasing depersonalization of services as the bureaucracies get larger, more entrenched, and less and less open to change. There is, as yet, no method of intelligent and deliberate change to which all groups at interest will agree. Thus we continue to revert to political power to force change if a consensus can be mustered at the polls.

So I fall back on my recommendations which it seems are congenial to the American political and social system. At relatively modest cost, with a maximum of equity, and a maximum of flexibility of operation and financing, I would like to see the following evolve as a national health policy for the indefinite future. For the sake of equity, and to test our humaneness as a society, a systematic attempt should be made to get comprehensive services to the poor by two chief methods. One is a generous government subsidy to buy health insurance policies from the current insurance agencies of all types to facilitate entry to the "mainstream" of American medicine on the part of the poor who are aggressive enough to seek it. Parallel to this subsidy of health insurance policies I would set up massive incentive subsidies to hospitals and medical centers to provide services to those in poverty areas. With this second method, the poor would then have options too.

For the employed segment of the population—an overwhelming proportion of whom already carry some type of health insurance in connection with their employment—I would suggest a federal health insurance system to cover high-cost episodes of given magnitudes, say above $15,-000. New taxes would be quite minimal. The poor would get comprehensive services for nothing and with options. The employed and earning segment of the population would be rid of the fear of family financial catastrophe.

Organizationally, the entire population should be given options to enroll in the Blue Cross : Blue Shield Plans, private insurance companies, the group practice plan, and the comprehensive physician fee-for-service plans. The employed segment of the population should be given options for the level of benefits and method of delivery. The government should pay the catastrophic portion of the premium, and the employee can pay according to whatever range of services he wishes to afford.

Underpinning this proposal and an integral part of it, is the recommendation that government and private sources, predominantly government, accelerate massively the training of more physicians, nurses, dentists, and related technical personnel. Delivery methods should be

innovated to compete in an environment of relative abundance of personnel and facilities. This country can afford this philosophy of expansive-
ness for the entire population and minimize the differences of care for the
poor and the comfortable.

The trend toward increasingly official planning bodies will likely lead
to a tight system not desired in the American context. Some planning is
still needed on a voluntary basis to avoid the gross examples of duplication and excess use of service. No central planning body knows how to
determine adequacy of facilities and personnel; hence a health system
generously proportioned is preferred rather than reliance on spurious
specificity and specifications. The great range of the number of general
hospital beds to population in the three countries supports this
observation—four beds per 1000 population in the United States and six
in Sweden.

Still, after having said all this, some sort of a muddled system and sub-
systems will evolve that will be changed in small detail from election to
election. Viable private and public sector interrelationships will not be
clearly thought through in order to maximize flexibility and funding,
but, then, this is the price the United States is willing to pay for an open
system. Our tripartite division of powers—legislative, administrative,
judicial—complicated by a federation of states, sets the stage for a very
freewheeling method of policy formulation. The parliamentary systems of
Great Britain and Sweden and the absence in both countries of a federation of relatively autonomous states makes for tidier policy development,
certainly by the time debate takes place in the respective legislative bodies.

While these recommendations are being written the usual supermarket
variety of proposals for some form of national health insurance are being
introduced in Congress. They range from a highly structured, centrally
financed, centrally directed by financial leverage to one that simply em-
ploys the federal income tax mechanism to assist the poor in buying
health insurance according to some defined minimum, leaving the current structure of delivering services essentially intact. Neither extreme is
likely to be adopted. My recommendations flow from assessment of what
is politically feasible, financially acceptable, and reasonably equitable in
the context of the American political and social system. Furthermore, it
is assumed that recommendations are reasonably acceptable to the providers. There is no necessary belief in the status quo because an arrangement is being suggested that is essentially dynamic and should be responsive to consumers when they have options. It would thus seem that these
recommendations embody a belief that the delivery system can in the
long haul change as consumers and providers evolve together in shaping

a variety of delivery systems to fit the various conditions of this large and variegated country. No one is being pushed around much. It is obvious that these recommendations may resemble proposals already being discussed. This is coincidental, but should be pointed out nevertheless. The concept of a national health service is one that fits the particular social, political, and economic system at a particular time with due regard for cost and equity. Apparently a few politicians and their advisors have arrived at the same conclusion intuitively. Such is the state of the art.

The English and Swedish systems will continue basically as they are. The English system may become even more highly structured by abolishing the tripartite divisions and centralizing administration and funding even more, the assumption being that these result in great rationalization of services. The Swedes will probably have the most generously distributed hospital and medical system in the world as long as the County Councils have no other responsibility and are given, as they now have, the commensurate taxing power.

The United States in the foreseeable future will not, of course, approximate the equity of the English and Swedish systems for the many reasons described in this book. Nevertheless, the United States will probably achieve a reasonable minimum of service for those of low income although more of a gap will remain in care provided and amenities than is true in Britain and Sweden. This very lack of worry about pure equity will keep the United States health services relatively more dynamic, though some may argue that this is too big a price to pay. Each society expresses its concept of distributive justice through the political process. Sweden and England have clearly revealed their concept of distributive justice; the United States will be in the process of revealing its concept during the coming decade. If this country will fund a generously proportioned system of options for the well-off and comprehensive services for the badly off, it can have both dynamism and equity.

COMPARATIVE TABLES RELATING TO HEALTH CARE IN THE UNITED STATES, SWEDEN, AND ENGLAND AND WALES

DEMOGRAPHIC DATA

FINANCING

PERSONNEL AND FACILITIES

VITAL STATISTICS

DEMOGRAPHIC DATA

TABLE A1   POPULATION AND POPULATION DENSITY

Demographic Characteristics	United States[a]	Sweden	England and Wales
Land area in square miles	3,022,387	174,000	58,000
Population			
1950	150,697,000	7,014,000	43,758,000
1960	179,323,000	7,495,000	46,072,000
1970	202,143,000	8,013,696	48,827,000
Population density per square mile			
1950	50	40	754
1960	59	43	794
1970	67	46	842

A BREAKDOWN OF THE LOWEST AND HIGHEST DENSITIES IN EACH COUNTRY

Country	Most Dense[b]		Least Dense	
	Name of Area	Density per Square Mile	Name of Area	Density per Square Mile
United States	New York City	25,966	Wyoming	3.2
Sweden	Stockholm	10,691	Norrbottens	7.8
England and Wales	London conurbation	11,339	Wales	333.8

Sources. United States: Bureau of the Census (1968), pp. 10–12, 17, 21. Sweden: National Central Bureau of Statistics (1968), pp. 29–30; (1970), pp. 26–27. For Sweden the density of population is given in square kilometers and has been converted to square miles by dividing by 0.386. England and Wales: Central Statistical Office (1965), pp. 1, 7, 11. Department of Health and Social Security (1971), p. 2.

[a]Excludes Alaska and Hawaii. Population based upon April 1 official census figures.

[b]The majority of the population in all three countries is located in the cities: 69.9 percent in the United States, 77.4 percent in Sweden, and 79.2 percent in England and Wales.

FINANCING

TABLE A2   SOURCES OF FINANCING FOR THE HEALTH CARE
SYSTEM

Source	United States	Sweden	England and Wales
1950			
Private			
Consumer direct	57.1%	15.7%	15.4%
Insurance	9.0	6.3[a]	—
Philanthropy	4.0	—	—
Other[b]	2.1	—	—
	72.2%	22.0%	15.4%
Public			
Federal	13.3%	25.8%	78.9%
Local	14.5	52.2	5.7
	27.8%	78.0%	84.6%
Total	100%	100%	100%
1965			
Private			
Consumer direct	44.1%	15.0%	14.7%
Insurance	25.1	—	0.5
Philanthropy	3.5	—[a]	—
Other	2.4	—	—
	75.1%	15.0%	15.2%
Public			
Federal	12.4%	19.8%	79.4%
Local	12.5	65.2	5.4
	24.9%[c]	85.0%	84.8%
Total	100%	100%	100%

Sources. United States: 1950 data from Reed and Hanft (1966); 1965 data from
Rice and Cooper (1968). Sweden: 1950 data from National Board of Health
(1952); 1965 data *op. cit.* (1967); private expenditure data developed from the
sources given above based on information contained in Albinsson (1965). England and Wales: 1950 data on private expenditures from Paige and Jones
(1966), pp. 125, 141; all other data for 1950 from Abel-Smith and Titmuss
(1956), pp. 24–47. 1965 data on private insurance from Mencher (1968), pp. 16,

TABLE A3   SOURCES OF FINANCING FOR THE HEALTH CARE
SYSTEM IN THE UNITED STATES

	1950	1965	1969[a]
Private			
Consumer direct	57.1%	44.1%	35.0%
Insurance	9.0	25.1	19.0
Philanthropy	4.0	3.5	8.0
Other	2.1	2.4	
	72.2%	75.1%	62.0%
Public			
Federal	13.3%	12.4%	25.5%
Local	14.5	12.5	12.5
	27.8%	24.9%	38.0%
Total	100%	100%	100%

Source. Social Security Administration (1969).

[a] Although the table shows the shifting financing of all health care from the private to the public sector in the last four years, this is not the whole story. It should be remembered that private and public expenditures are concentrated in different subsections of the health care system:

Area	Private	Public	All Expenditures
Professional personnel	82%	18%	$17.2 billion
Hospital care	50	50	22.6 billion
Drugs and appliances	97	3	7.7 billion
Nursing home care	18	82	2.2 billion
Construction	60	40	2.4 billion
Medical research	21	79	1.9 billion
Other	41	59	6.3 billion
Total	62%	38%	$60.3 billion

23; data on private expenditures from Paige and Jones (1966). All other data from Ministry of Health (1968), pp. 76–77.

[a] Before 1955 sickness insurance funds were voluntary. In 1955 they were made compulsory under a program administered by the Swedish government.

[b] Industrial health services and expenditures for construction made from capital funds.

[c] This picture has, of course, changed with the introduction of Medicare and Medicaid in 1966. Medicare is entirely federally financed, while Medicaid is shared between federal and local governments. From 24.9 percent of total expenditure in 1965 the state and federal share jumped to 37.1 percent in 1968.

TABLE A4   TOTAL COST OF THE HEALTH CARE SYSTEM

Year	United States Amount	Percent Increase	Sweden Amount	Percent Increase	England and Wales Amount	Percent Increase
1950	$12.8 billion	—	SK 848 million	—	£ 583 million	—
1955	$18.0 billion	41	SK 1676 million	98	£ 723 million	24
1960	$27.0 billion	111	SK 2804 million	231	£1075 million	84
1965	$40.9 billion	220	SK 5537 million	553	£1400 million	140
1968	$53.7 billion	320	SK 9695 million	1043	£1858 million	219
			Per Capita			
1950	$ 84.06	—	SK 121	—	£13.3	—
1955	$108.48	29	SK 231	91	£16.3	23
1960	$149.43	78	SK 375	210	£23.5	77
1965	$210.17	132	SK 716	492	£29.2	120
1968	$269.43	221	SK 1225	912	£34.5	159

Sources. United States: 1950, 1955, 1960 derived from Reed and Hanft (1966); 1965, from Rice and Cooper (1968) 1968 from Bureau of the Census (1971), p. 62. Sweden: 1950 from National Board of Health (1956), p. 77; 1955 *ibid.* (1959), pp. 80–81; 1960 *ibid.* (1962), p. X; 1965, *ibid.* (1968), p. XIII. 1968 *ibid.* (1971), p. 94. England and Wales: 1950, 1955, 1960 from Paige and Jones (1966), derived from pp. 125 and 141. 1965 from Ministry of Health (1968). 1968 from Department of Health and Social Security Digest (1971), pp. 6–7. All years include expenditures outside of the National Health Service.

TABLE A5 INFLATION IN THE ECONOMY, 1950 TO 1970

Year	Percent Increase in Consumer Price Index		
	United States	Sweden	England and Wales
1950	—	—	—
1955	11	32	21
1960	23	57	36
1965	31	88	62
1966	35	100	68
1967	40	109	73
1968	45	113	81
1969	52	119	91
1970	61	a	a

Sources. United States: Bureau of the Census (1971), derived from p. 339. Sweden: National Central Bureau of Statistics (1970), derived from p. 212. England and Wales: Central Statistical Office (1965), derived from p. 319, updated to 1966, *ibid.* (1969), p. 354. 1967–1970 from Central Statistical Office (1970), derived from p. 85.

a Not available.

TABLE A6 TOTAL COST OF THE HEALTH CARE SYSTEM AS A
PERCENT OF NATIONAL INCOME[a]

| | Percent of National Income | | |
Year	United States	Sweden	England and Wales[b]
1950	5.3	3.2	4.4
1955	5.4	4.0	3.9
1960	6.5	4.9	4.3
1965	7.3	5.5	4.6
1966	7.4	6.5	4.9
1967	7.6	7.3	5.1
1968	7.5	8.1	5.2
1969	7.8	c	5.3
1970	8.4	c	5.6

Sources of national income data. United States: Bureau of the Census (1971), p.
311. Sweden: National Central Bureau of Statistics (1968), p. 355. *ibid.* (1970),
p. 338. England and Wales: Office of Health Economics (1971).
[a] Gross national product less capital consumption allowances and indirect business tax and nontax liability. For Sweden this is defined as gross domestic product at factor cost.
[b] These figures exclude private expenditures made outside of the National Health Service. Including outside expenditures would have the effect of raising the percent by about one half a percentage point.
[c] Not available.

TABLE A7 PERCENT INCREASE IN NATIONAL INCOME[a]

Year	United States	Sweden	England and Wales
1950	—	—	—
1955	37	57	44
1960	72	115	90
1965	133	280	162
1966	156	312	174
1968	220	377	203
1970	232	b	258

Sources. See Table A6.
[a] Gross national product less capital consumption allowances and indirect business tax and nontax liability. For Sweden this is defined as gross domestic product at factor cost.
b Not available.

Component of Care	United States	Sweden	England and Wales
	1950		
Hospital care	29.7%	47.3%	41.7%
Physicians [a]	21.9	13.7	16.0
Dentists	7.8	7.1	6.5
Other professional services	3.1	—	—
Drugs	13.3	6.7	15.5
Eyeglasses and appliances	3.9	—	3.1
Nursing homes	.8	3.9	3.9
Expenses for prepayment and administration	2.3	0.4	0.3
Public health	3.1	3.6	1.2
Other	7.0	8.5	8.4
Research and education	.8	2.4	—
Construction	6.3	6.4	3.4
Total	100.0%	100.0%	100.0%
	1965		
Hospital care	34.0%	46.9%	38.9%
Physicians [a]	21.5	13.9	13.1
Dentists	6.8	9.7	4.6
Other professional services	2.4	—	—
Drugs	11.7	8.3	19.0
Eyeglasses and appliances	2.9	—	1.4
Nursing home care	3.1	5.9	3.5
Expenses for prepayment and administration	3.1	0.4	1.0
Government public health activities	1.7	1.7	1.0
Other health services	4.4	3.2	12.4
Research and education	3.7	2.8	—
Construction	4.7	7.5	5.1
Total	100.0%	100.0%	100.0%

[a] Includes 10 percent of hospital expense in England and Wales and Sweden as adjustment for hospital-salaried physicians.

Sources. United States: 1950 from Reed and Hanft (1966); 1965 from Rice and Cooper (1968). Sweden: 1950 data from National Board of Health (1952); 1965 data *op. cit.* (1967); private expenditure data developed from the sources above based on information contained in Albinsson (1965). England and Wales: 1950 data on private expenditures from Paige and Jones (1966), pp. 125, 141; all other data for 1950 from Abel-Smith and Titmuss (1956), pp. 24–47. 1965 data on private insurance from Mencher (1968), pp. 16, 23; data on private expenditures from Paige and Jones (1966). All other data from Ministry of Health (1968), pp. 76–77.

TABLE A9   COMPARISON OF TOTAL EXPENDITURES OF THE HEALTH SERVICES SYSTEM IN THE UNITED STATES, SWEDEN, AND ENGLAND AND WALES

Subcomponent of Expenditure	United States	Sweden	England and Wales
	1950		
Actual expenditures, by source			
Private			
Consumer direct	$ 7.3 billion	SK 133 million	£ 90 million
Insurance	1.2 billion	53 million[c]	[o]
Philanthropy	0.4 billion	—	—
Other	0.3 billion[a]	—	—
Public			
Federal	1.7 billion	219 million	460 million
Local	1.9 billion	443 million	33 million
Total	$12.8 billion	SK 848 million	£583 million
Actual expenditures, by type			
Hospital care	$ 3.8 billion	SK 401 million[d]	£243 million[p]
Physician service	2.8 billion	116 million[e]	93 million[q]
Dentist service	1.0 billion	60 million[f]	38 million
Other professional service	0.4 billion	[g]	[g]
Drugs	1.7 billion	57 million[h]	90 million[r]
Eyeglasses and appliances	0.5 billion	[g]	18 million
Nursing home care	0.1 billion	34 million	23 million
Expenses for prepayment and administration	0.3 billion	3 million[i, j]	2 million
Government public health activities	0.4 billion	31 million[k]	7 million
Other health services	0.9 billion[b]	72 million[l]	49 million[s]
Research and education	0.1 billion	20 million[m, j]	[t]
Construction	0.8 billion	54 million[n]	20 million
Total	$12.8 billion	SK 848 million	£583 million

Sources of 1950 data. United States: Reed and Hanft (1966). Sweden: Based on 1950 data contained in National Board of Health (1952). For the development of private expenditures, see Table A2. See footnotes for extensive adjustments made to these tables. England and Wales: Private insurance data from Mencher (1968), pp. 16, 23. Data on private expenditures and on total expenditures from Paige and Jones (1966), pp. 125, 141. All other data from Abel-Smith and Titmuss (1956), pp. 24–47. See footnotes for adjustments made to these data.

Subcomponent of Expenditure	United States	Sweden	England and Wales
	1955		
Actual expenditures, by source			
Private			
Consumer direct	$ 9.5 billion	SK 240 million	£126 million
Insurance	2.9 billion	c	1 million
Philanthropy	0.6 billion	—	—
Other	0.3 billion[a]	—	—
Public			
Federal	2.1 billion	373 million	574 million
Local	2.6 billion	1063 million	22 million
Total	$18.0 billion	SK 1676 million	£723 million
Actual expenditures, by type			
Hospital care	$ 5.9 billion	SK 812 million[d]	£299 million[p]
Physician service	3.7 billion	204 million[e]	109 million[q]
Dentist service	1.5 billion	141 million[f]	29 million
Other professional service	0.6 billion	[g]	[g]
Drugs	2.4 billion	100 million[h]	118 million[r]
Eyeglasses and appliances	0.6 billion	[g]	8 million
Nursing home care	0.2 billion	73 million	29 million
Expenses for prepayment and administration	0.6 billion	5 million[i]	4 million[u]
Government public health activities	0.4 billion	43 million[k]	12 million
Other health services	1.2 billion[b]	163 million[l]	95 million[s]
Research and education	0.2 billion	33 million[m]	[t]
Construction	0.7 billion	102 million[n]	20 million
Total	$18.0 billion	SK 1676 million	£723 million

Sources of 1955 data. United States: Reed and Hanft (1966). Sweden: All public data from National Board of Health (1957). For the development of private expenditures see Table A2. See footnotes for extensive adjustments made to these data. England and Wales: Private insurance data from Mencher (1968). Data on private expenditures and on total expenditures from Paige and Jones (1966). All other data from Feldstein, Martin, unpublished material. See footnotes for adjustments made to these data.

Subcomponent of Expenditure	United States	Sweden	England and Wales
	1960		
Actual expenditures, by source			
Private			
Consumer direct	$13.2 billion	SK 435 million	£ 178 million
Insurance	5.7 billion	—	4 million
Philanthropy	0.9 billion	—	—
Other	0.6 billion[a]	—	—
Public			
Federal	3.0 billion	601 million	824 million
Local	3.6 billion	1768 million	69 million
Total	$27.0 billion	SK 2804 million	£1075 million
Actual expenditures, by type			
Hospital care	$ 9.0 billion	SK 1202 million[d]	£ 445 million[p]
Physician service	5.7 billion	425 million[e]	135 million[q]
Dentist service	2.0 billion	261 million[f]	50 million
Other professional service	0.9 billion	[g]	[g]
Drugs	3.7 billion	233 million[h]	180 million[r]
Eyeglasses and appliances	0.8 billion	[g]	13 million
Nursing home care	0.5 billion	175 million	47 million
Expenses for prepayment and administration	0.9 billion	10 million[i]	7 million
Government public health activities	0.4 billion	56 million[k]	14 million
Other health services	1.5 billion[b]	176 million[l]	140 million[s]
Research and education	0.6 billion	70 million[m]	[t]
Construction	1.0 billion	196 million[n]	44 million
Total	$27.0 billion	SK 2804 million	£1075 million

Sources of 1960 data. United States: Reed and Hanft (1966). Sweden: All public data from National Board of Health (1962). For the development of private expenditures, see Table A2. See footnotes for extensive adjustments made to these data. England and Wales: Private insurance data from Mencher (1968). Data on private expenditures from Paige and Jones (1966). All other data from Central Statistical Office (1965), pp. 42, 43, 45, 53. See footnotes for adjustments made to these data.

TABLE A9 COMPARISON OF TOTAL EXPENDITURES OF THE
HEALTH SERVICES SYSTEM IN THE UNITED STATES,
SWEDEN, AND ENGLAND AND WALES (*Continued*)

Subcomponent of Expenditure	United States	Sweden	England and Wales
	1965		
Actual expenditures, by source			
Private			
Consumer direct	$18.0 billion	SK 833 million	£ 206 million
Insurance	10.3 billion	—	7 million
Philanthropy	1.4 billion	—	—
Other	1.0 billion[a]	—	—
Public			
Federal	5.1 billion	1098 million	1112 million
Local	5.1 billion	3606 million	75 million
Total	$40.9 billion	5537 million	£1400 million
Actual expenditures, by type			
Hospital care	$13.8 billion	SK 2583 million[d]	£ 545 million[p]
Physician service	8.8 billion	769 million[e]	183 million[q]
Dentist service	2.8 billion	535 million[f]	64 million[v]
Other professional service	1.0 billion	[g]	[g]
Drugs	4.8 billion	458 million[h]	267 million[r]
Eyeglasses and appliances	1.2 billion	[g]	19 million
Nursing home care	1.3 billion	327 million	49 million
Expenses for prepayment and administration	1.3 billion	21 million[i]	15 million
Government public health activities	.7 billion	93 million[k]	14 million
Other health services	1.8 billion[b]	179 million[l]	173 million[s]
Research and education	1.5 billion	159 million[m]	[t]
Construction	1.9 billion	413 million[n]	71 million
Total	$40.9 billion	SK 5537 million	£1400 million

222

Sources of 1965 data. United States: Rice and Cooper (1968). Sweden: All public data from National Board of Health (1967). For the development of private expenditures, see Table A2. See footnotes for extensive adjustments made to these data. England and Wales: Private insurance data from Mencher (1968). Data on private expenditures from Paige and Jones (1966). All other data from Ministry of Health (1968), pp. 76–77. See footnotes for adjustments made to these data.

[a] Industrial health services and expenditures for construction made from capital funds.

[b] Industrial health services, school health programs, expenses of voluntary health agencies, and certain small federal programs not classified elsewhere.

[c] Before 1955 sickness insurance funds were voluntary. In 1955 they were made compulsory under a program administered by the Swedish government.

[d] Includes private expenditure from voluntary sickness funds for 1950 as well as expenditure from compulsory sickness funds for 1955, 1960, and 1965. Excludes 10 percent for hospital physician salaries which are shown as part of physician services. Mental hospital costs were calculated using total patient days and a cost per patient day equivalent to that of the state mental hospitals. These costs are as follows: 1950—SK 143 million; 1955—SK 245 million; 1960—SK 405 million; 1965—758 million. Excludes investments in hospitals, which are shown under construction. Excludes homes for the chronic sick and nursing homes, which are shown under nursing homes.

[e] Includes 10 percent of hospital expenses for employed physicians as follows: 1950—SK 51 million; 1955—SK 90 million; 1960—SK 153 million; 1965—SK 323 million. Expenses for physicians in private practice were calculated by using sick fund expenditures as 60 percent of total expenditures for 1955, 1960, and 1965. For 1950 only, a breakdown of sick fund expenditures was unavailable, and physician expenditures were calculated using the 1955 ratio of salaried to private practice expenditures.

[f] See Table A12, footnote b.

[g] Included in other health services.

[h] See Table A12, footnote d. For 1950 only, drug expenditures are prorated, based on 1955 ratio of physician expenditures to drug expenditures.

[i] Expenses of the national government only.

[j] Estimated based on ratio to total expenses in 1955.

[k] Includes midwives, public health nursing, and maternal and child care.

[l] This is a residual category containing, among other things, health care expenditures on the military and a small amount of transportation expenses in connection with health care which it was impossible to separate.

[m] Education only.

[n] This construction figure (called "investments") is inflated by the unavoidable

inclusion of new equipment in already existing facilities and is thus not directly comparable to those of the United States and Great Britain.

^{n} £250,000.

^{p} Includes private expenditures as follows: 1950—£17 million; 1955—£20 million; 1960—£28 million; 1965—£35 million. Excludes 8 percent of total expenses, which are shown under nursing home care, and 10 percent for hospital physician salaries, which are shown under physician services.

^{q} Includes private expenditures as follows: 1950—£17 million; 1955—£20 million; 1960—£28 million; 1965—£35 million. Includes 10 percent of hospital expenses for physicians' salaries: 1950—£26 million; 1955—£34 million; 1960—£53 million; 1965—£60 million.

^{r} Includes private expenditures as follows: 1950—£51 million; 1955—£59 million; 1960—£85 million; 1965—£95 million. This category is not strictly drug expenses, since it includes a considerable amount of public expenditure for welfare foods (including but not limited to vitamins) which cannot be separated.

^{s} This very large category contains the following items which are distributed into other categories in the United States: outpatient mental health services, maternal and child care health services (including expenses of home delivery), ambulances, chiropodists, meals on wheels, visiting nurses. Certain unidentifiable miscellaneous items are also included.

^{t} Included in hospital expenses.

^{u} This item was unavailable in the data for this year and has been estimated by taking the midpoint between 1950 and 1960 expenditures.

^{v} For 1965 only, sufficient detail was available to allocate the salaries of hospital employed specialists to dentists as well as to physicians. With £62 million spent for specialist salaries and 20,000 MDs and 600 dentists employed by the hospitals, the expense was divided as follows: physicians—£60 million; dentists—£2 million. Ministry of Health, op. cit., pp. 162, 164, 188.

TABLE A10 YEAR-BY-YEAR COMPARISON OF THE INCREASE IN
COSTS OF THE TOTAL HEALTH CARE SYSTEM OF THE UNITED
STATES, SWEDEN, AND ENGLAND AND WALES, 1950 TO 1970

Year	United States Expenditure	Increase	Sweden Expenditure	Increase	England and Wales Expenditure	Increase
1950	$12.8 billion	100	SK 848 million	100	£583 million	100
1951	12.9 billion	101	1036 million	122	600 million	103
1952	13.9 billion	109	1236 million	146	629 million	108
1953	15.1 billion	118	1325 million	156	652 million	112
1954	16.2 billion	127	1525 million	180	675 million	116
1955	18.0 billion	141	1676 million	198	723 million	124
1956	19.1 billion	149	1923 million	227	795 million	136
1957	20.8 billion	163	2170 million	256	863 million	148
1958	22.3 billion	174	2370 million	279	915 million	157
1959	24.4 billion	191	2562 million	302	988 million	169
1960	27.0 billion	211	2804 million	331	1075 million	184
1961	28.9 billion	226	3120 million	368	1174 million	201
1962	31.4 billion	245	3578 million	422	1225 million	210
1963	33.6 billion	263	4089 million	482	1283 million	220
1964	37.5 billion	293	4676 million	551	1341 million	230
1965	40.9 billion	320	5537 million	653	1400 million	240
1966	45.4 billion	355	6750 million	796	1523 million	261
1967	49.6 billion	388	8119 million	957	1700 million	292
1968	53.7 billion	420	9695 million	1143	1858 million	319
1969	59.9 billion	468	a		2033 million	349
1970	67.2 billion	525	a		a	

Sources. United States: 1950, 1955, and 1960 from Reed and Hanft (1966); 1951–1954 and 1956–1959 from Reed and Rice (1962); 1965–1966 from Rice and Cooper (1968). 1967–1970 from Bureau of the Census (1971), p. 62. These latter figures exclude about two percent of expenditures included in the earlier series. Sweden: Public expenditures for 1950–1954 from National Board of Health (1956), p. 77; 1955–1959, *ibid.* (1959), pp. 80–81; 1960, *ibid.*, p. X; 1961–1966, *ibid.*, p. XIII. 1967–1968 *ibid.*, p. 94. For private expenditures, see Table A12. England and Wales: 1950–1962 from Paige and Jones (1966), pp. 125 and 141; 1963–1964—a uniform increase is assumed for these two years; 1965–1966 derived from Ministry of Health (1968). 1967–1969 derived from Department of Health and Social Security Digest (1971), pp. 6–7. All years include expenditures outside of those made by the National Health Service. About one quarter of these expenditures are reimbursements by patients to the NHS while approximately three quarters represent totally private expenditures.
a Not available

TABLE A11 INCREASE IN TOTAL HEALTH CARE EXPENDITURES, BY COMPONENT, IN THE UNITED STATES, SWEDEN, AND ENGLAND AND WALES, 1950 TO 1965; 1950 = 100

Subcomponent of Expenditure	United States				Sweden				England and Wales			
	1950	1955	1960	1965	1950	1955	1960	1965	1950	1955	1960	1965
By source												
Private												
Consumer-out-of-pocket	100	130	181	245	100	180	327	626	100	140	198	229
Insurance	100	241	475	858	100	403	730	1179	100	400	1600	2800
Philanthropy	100	150	225	350	—	—	—	—	—	—	—	—
Other	100	100	200	333	—	—	—	—	—	—	—	—
Public												
Federal	100	124	177	300	100	170	274	501	100	125	179	242
Local	100	137	189	268	100	192	312	673	100	67	209	227
By type												
Hospital care	100	155	237	350	100	202	300	644	100	123	183	224
Physician service	100	132	204	314	100	176	366	663	100	117	145	197
Dentist service	100	150	200	280	100	235	435	892	100	76	132	168
Other professional service					—	—	—	—	—	—	—	—
Drugs	100	150	225	250	100	176	409	804	—	131	200	297
Eyeglasses and appliances	100	141	218	282	—	—	—	—	100	44	72	106
Nursing home care	100	120	160	240	100	215	514	916	100	126	204	213
Expenses for prepayment and administration	100	200	300	433	100	167	333	700	100	200	350	750
Government public health activities	100	100	100	175	100	139	181	300	100	171	200	200
Other health services	100	133	167	200	100	226	244	249	100	194	286	353
Research and education	100	200	600	1500	100	165	350	795	—	—	—	—
Construction	100	88	125	238	100	189	363	765	100	100	220	855
Total	100	141	211	320	100	198	331	653	100	124	184	240

Source. Derived from Table A9.

226

TABLE A12   WORKSHEET FOR ESTIMATION OF PRIVATE EXPENDITURES ON HEALTH CARE IN SWEDEN, 1950 TO 1968 (IN MILLIONS OF KRONER)

		Private Expenditures					
	Total Public		Physi-	Drugs		Hospital	All Expendi- tures
Year	Expendi- ture[a]	Dental[b]	cian[c]	Pre- scribed[d]	Nonpre- scribed[e]	Care[f]	Combined
1950	SK 715	SK 40	SK 26	SK 57		SK 10	SK 848
1951	881	52	28	60		15	1036
1952	1046	69	31	70		20	1236
1953	1105	80	35	80		25	1325
1954	1280	84	41	90		30	1525
1955	1436	94	46	100			1676
1956	1647	109.	47	120			1923
1957	1856	126	48	140			2170
1958	2033	139	48	150			2370
1959	2180	159	99	55	69		2562
1960	2369	186	109	62	78		2804
1961	2642	198	116	73	91		3120
1962	3039	228	126	82	103		3578
1963	3458	294	141	87	109		4089
1964	3984	302	154	105	131		4676
1965	4704	380	178	122	153		5537
1966	5841	408	190	138	173		6750
1967	7037	488	228	163	203		8119
1968	8403	583	272	194	243		9695

[a] As reported in National Board of Health (1952–1971). Includes expenditures from sickness funds for all years.

[b] Since about a third of the dentists in Sweden are employed by the Public Health Service, the data shown for public expenditures for dental care are assumed to be about one third of total expenditures for dental care. (1950— 33.3%; 1955—33.3%; 1960—32%; 1965—29%). The other two thirds of this expenditure is therefore attributed to private out-of-pocket expenditure. The amount attributed to private dental care may be slightly understated, since some adults seen by Public Health Service dentists were paying patients but are not included in this figure.

[c] Based on a reimbursement from the sickness funds of about three quarters of the cost of seeing a general practitioner and one half the cost of seeing a specialist, a compromise figure of 60 percent reimbursement for physician care was arrived at. The remaining 40 percent of total expenditures of these items was

attributed to private expenditure. Prior to 1955 estimates only are available, based on the ratio pertaining in 1955 of salaried to nonsalaried physician expenditures.

[d] This item is shown separately from 1959–1966 only, based on an assumption of 50 percent reimbursement of drug expenses except for lifesaving drugs which are provided free. A compromise figure of 60 percent was arrived at and applied to drug reimbursement by the sickness funds. Prior to 1959, the data are estimates only and are included in a composite figure for prescription and non-prescription drugs.

[e] This item is paid for completely within the private sector. The United States cost ratio of two thirds prescription drugs to one third non prescription drugs was used here with the prescription drug cost obtained as explained in footnote d.

[f] Beginning in 1955, membership in a sickness fund became compulsory and these funds assumed the small out-of-pocket expenses previously associated with hospitalization. Before 1955 a small amount has been allowed for the minority of the population not covered by sickness funds on a voluntary basis. The small amount of extra amenity and private room hospital care is not included in these figures, which are therefore slightly understated.

TABLE A13   YEAR-BY-YEAR COMPARISON OF THE INCREASE
IN PER CAPITA COSTS OF THE TOTAL HEALTH CARE
SYSTEM IN THE UNITED STATES, SWEDEN, AND
ENGLAND AND WALES, 1950 TO 1968

	United States		Sweden		England and Wales	
Year	Per Capita Expenditure	Increase	Per Capita Expenditure	Increase	Per Capita Expenditure	Increase
1950	$ 84.06	100	SK 121	100	£13.3	100
1951	83.30	99	146	121	13.7	103
1952	88.23	105	173	143	14.3	108
1953	94.27	112	185	153	14.7	111
1954	99.37	118	211	174	15.2	114
1955	108.48	129	231	191	16.3	123
1956	113.08	135	263	217	17.8	134
1957	120.94	144	295	244	19.2	144
1958	127.52	152	320	264	20.3	153
1959	137.21	163	344	284	21.8	164
1960	149.43	178	375	310	23.5	177
1961	157.27	187	415	343	25.4	191
1962	168.22	200	473	391	26.2	197
1963	177.39	211	538	445	27.2	205
1964	195.19	232	610	504	28.2	212
1965	210.17	250	716	592	29.2	220
1966	230.55	274	864	714	31.5	237
1968	269.43	321	1225	1012	34.5	259

Sources. United States: Calculated from total expenditures as shown in Table A10 and total United States population including armed forces abroad from Bureau of the Census (1968). Sweden: Calculated from total expenditures as shown in Table A10 and total Swedish population from National Central Bureau of Statistics (1968). England and Wales: Calculated from total expenditures as shown in Table A10 and total population of England and Wales from Central Statistical Office (1965).

PERSONNEL AND FACILITIES

TABLE A14 INCREASE IN PER CAPITA EXPENDITURES FOR THE HEALTH CARE SYSTEM, 1950 TO 1965

Component of Expenditure	United States				Sweden				England and Wales			
	1950	1955	1960	1965	1950	1955	1960	1965	1950	1955	1960	1965
Hospital care	100	143	200	285	100	196	282	586	100	120	173	204
Physician services	100	122	172	246	100	165	335	582	100	119	138	181
Dentist services	100	138	169	219	100	211	389	767	100	78	122	144
Other professional services	100	138	190	196	100	—	—	—	100	—	—	—
Drugs	100	130	184	221	100	175	387	738	100	129	186	267
Eyeglasses and appliances	100	110	135	188	100	—	—	—	100	—	—	—
Nursing home care	100	183	421	1015	100	200	460	840	100	50	75	100
Expenses for prepayment and administration	100	183	253	338	100	175	325	675	100	140	200	200
Government public health activities	100	92	84	137	100	150	175	300	100	180	300	620
Other health services	100	123	140	157	100	220	240	230	100	150	150	150
Research and education	100	183	505	1173	100	167	300	700	100	191	282	327
Construction	100	80	106	186	100	175	325	663	100	100	200	300
Total	100	129	178	250	100	191	310	592	100	123	177	220

Sources. United States: 1950, 1955, 1960 from Reed and Hanft (1966); 1965 from Rice and Cooper (1968). Sweden: 1950 from National Board of Health (1956), p. 77; 1955 from *ibid.* (1959), pp. 80–81; 1960, *ibid.* (1962), p. X; 1965, *ibid.* (1968), p. XIII. Private expenditures developed as shown in Table A13. England and Wales: 1950, 1955, 1960 from Paige and Jones (1966), pp. 125 and 141. 1965 from Ministry of Health (1968). All years include expenditures outside of the National Health Service.

TABLE A15   PHYSICIANS (MDs) PER 100,000 POPULATION

Year	United States[a]	Sweden	England and Wales
1950	149	69	99
1955	150	78	108
1960	148	95	115
1967	158	117	119
1968	161	124	[b]

Sources. United States: NCHS, Health Resources Statistics (1972), p. 147. Sweden: National Board of Health (1969), p. 82. National Central Bureau of Statistics (1970), p. 270. England and Wales: Royal Commission on Medical Education (1968), p. 133.
[a] Includes osteopaths and inactive physicians.
[b] Comparable figure not available

TABLE A16   NURSES (RNs)[a] PER 100,000 POPULATION

Year	United States	Sweden[b]	England and Wales
1950	249	182	131
1955	254	231	158
1960	282	294	183
1967	325	335	215
1968	331	349	218

Sources. United States: NCHS, Health Resources Statistics (1972), p. 177. Sweden: National Board of Health (1969), p. 82. National Central Bureau of Statistics (1970), pp. 28, 270. England and Wales: Derived from Department of Health and Social Security Digest (1969), p. 24 and (1970) p. 31. A 9.3 percent adjustment has been made for RNs not attached to a hospital based on Paige and Jones (1966), p. 114. (1950—57,262; 1955—70,506; 1960—83,751; 1967—104,149; 1968—105,767.)
[a] Active nurses, including those working part-time. This amounts to about one quarter of the total in the United States and England and Wales. Data are not available for Sweden.
[b] Includes nurse-midwives—10 percent of the total in Great Britain and 5 percent in Sweden. In England and Wales all midwives are RNs. In Sweden, only two thirds of midwives are RNs.

TABLE A17 DENTISTS (DDSs) PER 100,000 POPULATION

Year	United States	Sweden	England and Wales
1950	57	49	22
1955	57	60	23
1960	56	68	23
1967	56	78	23
1968	57	79	24

Sources. United States: NCHS, Health Resources Statistics (1972), p. 75. This figure is pro-rated from 1970. Sweden: National Board of Health (1969), p. 82. National Central Bureau of Statistics (1970), p. 270. England and Wales: 1950, 1955, 1960 from Paige and Jones (1966), p. 47; 1967 from Department of Health and Social Security Digest (1969), p. 34, 1968 computed from *ibid.* (1971), pp. 2, 30, 44.

TABLE A18 DISTRIBUTION OF ACTIVE PHYSICIANS BY TYPE OF PRACTICE, 1967

	United States		Sweden		England and Wales	
Type of Care	Number	Percent	Number	Percent	Number	Percent
Patient care[a]						
General practice	68,306	23.2	3251	35.1	21,305	48.3
Specialties						
Medical	62,182	21.1	2413	26.1	6,071	13.8
Surgical	79,349	27.0	1588	17.2	8,924	20.2
Other	64,353	21.9	1188	12.9	6,695	15.8
		70.0		56.2		49.8
Total	274,190	93.2	8440	91.3	43,265	98.1
Nonpatient care	19,882	6.8	800	8.7	831	1.9
Total active physicians	294,072	100.0	9240	100.0	44,096	100.0

Sources. United States: American Medical Association (1968), p. 6, Table A. Sweden: National Board of Health (1969), pp. 82, 150. Physicians shown under nonpatient care are medical officers who give some patient care, particularly in rural areas. England and Wales: Department of Health and Social Security (1969), pp. 15, 26, 28. The nonpatient care category is composed of MDs on the

TABLE A19   DISTRIBUTION, BY SITE OF PRACTICE,
OF PHYSICIANS PROVIDING PATIENT CARE, 1967

	United States		Sweden		England and Wales	
Site of Practice	Number	Percent	Number	Percent	Number	Percent
Out of hospital	208,447	76	3080	36	21,305[a]	49
In hospital[b]	65,743	24	5360	64	21,960	51
Total	274,190	100	8440	100	43,265	100

Sources. United States: American Medical Association (1968), pp. 8, 10; in-hospital physicians include all nonfederal physicians with a hospital-based practice and those federal physicians who are with the Veteran's Administration. Sweden: National Board of Health (1969), pp. 42, 55, 56. England and Wales: See Table A18.

[a] Includes GP's working part-time in hospitals.
[b] Includes residents but not interns.

Regional Hospital Board Headquarters Staff, the mass radiography units and blood transfusion centers staff, and the following hospital specialists: social medicine, biochemistry, haematology, morbid anatomy, bacteriology, and blood transfusion. Note that the estimate of 44,096 active physicians is considerably lower than the 52,800 persons who reported themselves as physicians to the Bureau of the Census in Royal Commission on Medical Education (1968), p. 290. Therefore, this table does not agree with the physician-population ratios shown in Table A15 which were taken from Royal Commission on Medical Education (1968), p. 133.

[a] Includes residents but not interns.

TABLE A20   PERSONNEL PER PATIENT DAY—SHORT-TERM
GENERAL HOSPITALS

Year	United States	Sweden	England and Wales[a]
1950	1.78	1.31	1.51
1955	2.03	1.44	1.55
1960	2.26	1.36	1.77
1967	2.65	1.44	2.38
1968	2.72	1.63	[b]

Sources. United States: American Hospital Association (1970), p. 473. Sweden: National Board of Health (1969). Derived from pp. 25 and 42. (1971). Derived from pp. 27 and 59. Personnel per 100 beds divided by percent occupancy. England and Wales: Ministry of Health (1969), p. 42.

[a]Because of the methods of bookkeeping of the National Health Service, these figures are not available for short-term hospitals. Instead, figures for all hospitals combined have been calculated (1950—0.89 personnel per patient day; 1955—0.91; 1960—1.04; 1967—1.40). The ratio of personnel per patient day in short-term general hospitals to personnel per patient day in all hospitals was then found for the United States (1.9 to 1) and for Sweden (1.5 to 1), and the midpoint (1.7 to 1) was taken for England and Wales, giving the figures shown in the table.

[b]Comparable figure not available.

TABLE A21   GENERAL HOSPITAL BEDS PER 1000 POPULATION

Year	United States	Sweden	England and Wales
1950	3.3	5.7	5.0
1955	3.5	5.8	4.7
1960	3.6	5.9	4.5
1965	3.9	5.9	4.3
1967	4.0	5.8	4.3
1968	4.0	5.9	4.2

Sources. United States: American Hospital Association (1970), p. 473. Sweden: National Board of Health (1971), pp. 48–49. General Hospital beds plus epidemic care and maternity beds. England and Wales: Department of Health and Social Security Digest (1971), p. 56 (nonpsychiatric, excluding geriatric and the chronic sick).

TABLE A22   ALL HOSPITAL BEDS PER 1000 POPULATION

Year	United States	Sweden	England and Wales
1950	9.6	14.1	10.4
1955	9.7	14.9	10.5
1960	9.2	15.6	10.5
1965	8.8	16.0	9.8
1967	8.4	16.0	9.7
1968	8.3	16.3	9.6

Sources. United States: American Hospital Association (1970), p. 472. Sweden: National Board of Health (1971), pp. 48–49. England and Wales: Department of Health and Social Security Digest (1971), p. 56.

TABLE A23   DISTRIBUTION OF GENERAL HOSPITAL BEDS BY AREA WITHIN EACH COUNTRY

		General Hospital Beds per 1000 Population			
		Highest		Lowest	
Country	Average Number	Area	Number	Area	Number
United States (1968)	4.0	District of Columbia	6.2	Maryland[a]	3.1
Sweden (1960)	4.9	Urban areas	6.0	Svealand region, excluding cities	4.0
England and Wales (1967)	4.3	Liverpool region	5.1	East Anglian region	2.7

Sources. United States: American Hospital Association (1969), computed from pp. 480–491. Sweden: Statens Öffentliga Utredningar (1963), p. 145. Excludes maternity beds, contagious disease beds, and certain other general hospital beds. England and Wales: Department of Health and Social Security (1969), pp. 44–45. Excludes maternity beds.
[a]Technically, Alaska, which is not on the United States mainland, has the lowest rate—2.1. Hawaii also has a rate lower than Maryland's.

TABLE A24   AVERAGE LENGTH OF STAY—SHORT-TERM GENERAL HOSPITALS

Year	United States	Sweden[a]	England and Wales
1950	8.1	15.8	—
1955	7.7	14.8	—
1960	7.6	13.8	15.0
1965	7.8	12.6	12.7
1967	8.3	12.1	11.9
1968	8.4	11.9	11.6

Sources. United States: American Hospital Association (1970), p. 473. Sweden: Calculated from National Board of Health (1971), calculated from pp. 48–49. In all tables concerning general hospitals in Sweden, the figures include general hospital care, epidemic care, and maternity care. England and Wales: Department of Health and Social Security Digest (1971), p. 57.
[a]Excludes epidemic and maternity care which would reduce length of stay by about 0.5 days.

TABLE A25   ADMISSIONS TO GENERAL HOSPITALS PER 1000 POPULATION

Year	United States	Sweden	England and Wales
1950	109.7	113.1	63.8
1955	116.6	117.5	—
1960	127.6	122.0	84.0
1965	136.4	132.5	93.7
1967	136.4	135.0	96.2
1968	136.9	137.7	98.2

Sources. United States: American Hospital Association (1970), p. 473. Sweden: National Board of Health (1971), pp. 48–49. General hospital admissions plus epidemic and maternity admissions. England and Wales: Department of Health and Social Security Digest (1971), p. 56 (nonpsychiatric, excluding geriatric and the chronic sick).

TABLE A26   ADMISSION TO PSYCHIATRIC HOSPITALS PER 1000 POPULATION

Year	United States[a]	Sweden	England and Wales
1950	3.2	—	1.8
1955	3.2	—	2.5
1960	3.3	5.6	3.2
1965	3.8	9.0	3.8
1967	4.2	10.4	4.0
1968	4.6	11.0	4.1

Sources. United States: American Hospital Association (1970), p. 472. Federal psychiatric hospital data hand-tabulated from ibid. (1969), pp. 18–237. National Institutes of Mental Health (1968), p. III–38. Sweden: National Board of Health (1971), pp. 48–49. Total mentally ill care plus care of mentally retarded and epileptics. England and Wales: Department of Health and Social Security Digest (1971), derived from p. 56.

[a] For 1967 the admissions breakdown was as follows: nonfederal psychiatric hospitals, 59%; psychiatric units in general hospitals, 34%; federal hospitals, 7%. This percentage distribution has been applied to the admissions to nonfederal psychiatric hospitals for all other years.

TABLE A27   ADMISSIONS TO ALL TYPES OF HOSPITALS PER 1000 POPULATION

Year	United States	Sweden	England and Wales
1950	121.7	120.6	67.4
1955	128.5	126.2	—
1960	139.0	133.8	90.4
1965	148.1	146.0	100.9
1967	148.4	152.8	103.6
1968	149.3	162.8	106.0

Sources. United States: American Hospital Association (1970), p. 472. Sweden: National Board of Health (1971), pp. 48–49. England and Wales: Department of Health and Social Security Digest (1971), p. 56.

TABLE A28 HOSPITAL DAYS PER 1000 POPULATION—
GENERAL HOSPITALS

Year	United States	Sweden	England and Wales
1950	890	1630	—
1955	900	1600	—
1960	970	1600	1260
1965	1070	1550	1205
1967	1130	1554	1132
1968	1154	1569	1132

Sources. United States: Derived from American Hospital Association (1970), p. 473. Sweden: National Board of Health (1971), pp. 48–49. General hospital days plus epidemic and maternity admissions. England and Wales: Department of Health and Social Security Digest (1971), derived from p. 56.

TABLE A29 HOSPITAL DAYS PER 1000 POPULATION—
MENTAL HOSPITALS

Year	United States[a]	Sweden	England and Wales
1950	1639	—	—
1955	1650	—	—
1960	1527	2329	1606
1965	1279	2204	1424
1967	1122	2153	1387
1968	1082	2177	1314

Sources. United States: American Hospital Association (1970), p. 472. Federal psychiatric data hand-tabulated from *ibid.* (1969) pp. 18–237. National Institutes of Mental Health (1968), p. III–38. Sweden: National Board of Health (1971), pp. 48–49. Total mentally ill care plus care of mentally retarded and epileptics. England and Wales: Department of Health and Social Security Digest (1971), derived from p. 56.

[a] For 1967 the breakdown of hospital days was as follows: nonfederal psychiatric hospitals, 90%; psychiatric units in general hospitals, 2%; and federal hospitals, 8%. This percentage distribution has been applied to the days for nonfederal psychiatric hospitals for all other years.

TABLE A30   HOSPITAL DAYS PER 1000 POPULATION—
TOTAL HOSPITALS

Year	United States	Sweden	England and Wales
1950	3010	—	3320
1955	2980	—	3300
1960	2840	4903	3270
1965	2660	4876	3030
1967	2550	4865	2957
1968	2524	4957	2884

Sources. United States: Derived from American Hospital Association (1970), p. 472. Sweden: National Board of Health (1971), pp. 48–49. England and Wales: Department of Health and Social Security Digest (1971), derived from p. 56.

TABLE A31 ANNUAL USE OF THE HEALTH CARE SYSTEM
BY THE ENTIRE POPULATION

Country	Percent of Population Seeing a Physician	Average Number of Physician Visits per Year	Percent of Population Admitted to a General Hospital	Percent Using Prescribed Drugs	Average Number of Prescriptions Filled	Percent of Population Seeing a Dentist	Average Number of Dentist Visits per Year
United States	68	4.3	10.0	43	4.7	38	1.4
Sweden	69	2.5	8.5	46	5.8	37[b]	0.4[c]
England and Wales	66	5.9	6.6[a]	62	4.5	43[b]	—

Sources. United States: physician care for 1966–1967 from NCHS, Series 10, Number 49, pp. 3, 38. Hospital care for 1965–1966 from NCHS, Series 10, Number 50, p. 2. Percent using prescribed drugs for 1963 from Andersen and Anderson (1967), p. 5. Average number of prescriptions filled for 1964–1965 from NCHS, Series 10, Number 39, calculated from pp. 17, 34. Percent of population seeing a dentist for 1963 from Andersen and Anderson (1967), p. 46. Average number of dentist visits per year for 1968 from NCHS, *Monthly Vital Statistics Report*, Vol. 18, No. 9, (1969), p. 1. Sweden: All data are for 1963 from Andersen, Smedby, and Anderson (1970), Tables 6, 9, 10, with the exception of average number of prescriptions filled, which is for 1967 from National Board of Health (1969), p. 78. England and Wales: Percent of population seeing a physician and average number of visits for 1964 from Cartwright (1967), p. 25. The general practitioner visits figure of 5.0 cited on p. 25 has been increased by the 0.94 outpatient attendances at hospitals on p. 130. Percent using prescribed drugs calculated from Ibid, p. 29. Average number of prescriptions filled from Department of Health and Social Security (1969), p. 55. Population seeing a dentist for 1968 from Department of Health and Social Security (1970), calculated from pp. 152–153. Average number of dental visits per year for 1968 from Department of Health and Social Security (1969), p. 49.

[a] Calculated by finding the ratio of single admissions to all admissions for the United States (0.73) and Sweden (0.65) and applying the midpoint (0.69) to all admissions for England and Wales.

[b] Excludes children under 16.

[c] Courses of treatment; actual number of dental visits was probably somewhat higher.

VITAL STATISTICS

TABLE A32   PERCENT OF PREMATURE BIRTHS[a]

United States (1964)	
White	7.1
Nonwhite	13.9
Total	8.1
Sweden (1968)	5.0
England and Wales (1968)	6.6

Sources. United States: NCHS, Series 21, No. 11 (1967), p. 25. Sweden: National Board of Health (1971). Calculated from p. 118. England and Wales: Department of Health and Social Security (1969), p. 110.

[a] Defined as birth of a live baby weighing less than 5½ pounds (2500 grams).

TABLE A33   PERCENT OF LIVE BIRTHS OCCURRING IN THE HOSPITAL

United States (1967)	98.5
Sweden (1967)	99.9
England and Wales (1968)	80.6

Sources. United States: NCHS, *Monthly Vital Statistics Report,* Vol. 18, No. 11. Sweden: National Board of Health (1969), p. 14. England and Wales: Department of Health and Social Security (1969), p. 77.

TABLE A34   MATERNAL MORTALITY PER 10,000
LIVE BIRTHS

Year	United States			Sweden	England and Wales
	White	Nonwhite	Total		
1930	60.0	120.0	66.0	a	42.4
1957	3.1	12.5	4.1	3.6	4.8
1966	2.0	7.2	2.9	1.1	2.6
1967	2.0	7.0	2.8	a	2.0
1968	1.7	6.4	2.5	a	2.4
1969	a	a	2.7	a	1.9

Sources. United States: Bureau of the Census (1968), p. 51. Sweden: 1957 from Lerner and Anderson (1963), p. 135; 1966 from National Board of Health (1968), p. 99. England and Wales: 1930 from Central Statistical Office (1965), p. 36; 1957 and 1966 from Department of Health and Social Security Digest (1969), p. 77, 1967–1969 from *ibid.* (1971), p. 2.

[a] Data not available.

TABLE A35   LEGAL ABORTIONS

United States	1966 (old law)	One for every 2000 live births nationwide
	1969 (new laws in 12 states)	One for every 170 live births nationwide
	1971 (legal abortion for any reason in New York State)	One for every 7 live births nationwide
Sweden	1965	One for every 20 live births
	1968	One for every 10 live births
England and Wales	1965 (old law)	One for every 194 live births
	1969 (new law)	One for every 14 live births
	1970 (revision of new law)	One for every 10 live births nationwide

Sources. United States: Medical World News, (1972) p. 15. Sweden: 1965 from National Board of Health (1967), p. 104; 1968 from Diggory (1970), p. 291. England and Wales: Diggory (1970), pp. 289, 291, Department of Health and Social Security Annual Report (1971), p. 66.

TABLE A36   DECLINE IN THE INFANT MORTALITY RATE

| Year | United States | | | Sweden | England and Wales |
	White	Nonwhite	Total		
1950	—	—	—	—	—
1960	14.6%	2.9%	11.0%	21.0%	30.6%
1965	19.8%	9.4%	15.4%	36.7%	39.5%
1967	26.5%	19.3%	24.3%	38.6%	41.4%
1968	28.3%	22.5%	25.3%	38.1%	41.7%

Source. Derived from Table 25 in the text.

TABLE A37   DEATH RATES PER 1000 POPULATION, 1965

Country	Crude		Age-Adjusted[a]
United States		9.4	9.4
White	9.4		9.1
Nonwhite	9.6		11.9
Sweden		10.1	8.2
England and Wales		11.5	8.9

[a]Based on 1967 United States resident population as shown in Bureau of the Census (1968), p. 10.

TABLE A38   LIFE EXPECTANCY AT BIRTH, 1965

United States		70.2
White	71.0	
Nonwhite	64.1	
Sweden		73.7
England and Wales		71.1

Sources. United States: Bureau of the Census (1968), p. 53. Sweden: National Central Bureau of Statistics (1968), calculated from p. 79. England and Wales: Central Statistical Office (1965), calculated from p. 38.

TABLE A39   REDUCTIONS IN AGE-SPECIFIC MORTALITY, 1940 TO 1966

	Deaths per 1000 Population								
	United States			Sweden			England and Wales		
Age	1940	1966	Percent Reduction	1940	1966	Percent Reduction	1940	1966	Percent Reduction
Under 1	54.9	23.3	63	38.9	12.7	67	52.3	19.2	63
1– 4	2.9	0.9	69	2.6	0.7	73	3.5	0.8	77
5– 9	1.1	0.4	64	0.9	0.4	56	1.5	0.4	73
10–14	1.0	0.4	60	0.9	0.3	67	1.0	0.3	70
15–19	1.7	1.0	41	1.7	0.7	59	1.8	0.7	61
20–24	2.4	1.3	46	2.7	0.8	70	2.4	0.7	71
25–29	2.8	1.4	50	2.5	0.7	72	2.5	0.8	68
30–34	3.4	1.7	50	2.6	1.0	62	2.7	1.0	63
35–39	4.4	2.4	45	2.9	1.5	48	3.4	1.5	56
40–44	6.1	3.7	39	3.8	2.2	42	4.6	2.6	43
45–49	8.7	5.8	33	5.7	3.3	42	6.8	4.3	37
50–54	12.8	9.1	29	8.2	5.3	35	10.5	7.3	30
55–59	18.6	14.0	24	12.2	8.2	17	15.6	11.9	24
60–64	26.8	20.5	24	18.6	14.0	25	24.3	19.6	19
65–69	39.2	31.7	19	30.3	23.5	22	37.5	31.3	17
70–74	61.1	46.5	24	51.7	39.9	23	60.9	48.7	20
75–79	94.8	68.2	28	87.9	69.5	21	96.5	77.5	20
80–84	145.6	105.8	27	149.6	114.8	23	148.2	124.0	16
85 and over	235.7	200.5	15	265.3	207.3	22	245.1	219.1	11

Sources. United Nations (1951), pp. 388, 398; *ibid.* (1968), pp. 416, 424.

TABLE A40   THE LOWEST AGE-SPECIFIC DEATH RATES
RECORDED IN WESTERN COUNTRIES, LATE 1960s

Age	Country with Lowest Rate	Rate [a]
Under 1	Sweden	12.7
1–4	Sweden	0.7
5–9	Belgium, Denmark, France, Hungary, Sweden, England and Wales, Scotland, Australia, New Zealand, United States	0.4
10–14	Denmark, France, Hungary, Sweden, England and Wales	0.3
15–19	Ireland	0.5
20–24	Denmark, Netherlands, Norway, England and Wales	0.7
25–29	Netherlands, Sweden	0.7
30–34	Norway, Sweden, England and Wales	1.0
35–39	Greece, Netherlands	1.3
40–44	Greece	2.1
45–49	Greece, Sweden	3.3
50–54	Greece	5.1
55–59	Greece, Sweden	8.2
60–64	Greece	13.4
65–69	Norway	23.2
70–74	Greece	36.4
75–79	Albania	59.1
80–84	Albania	75.8
85 and over	Albania	107.0

Source. United Nations (1968), pp. 420–425.

[a] Excludes countries with less than one million population because of the small number of deaths in some age categories. If it were not for this exclusion Iceland would have the lowest death rate in six categories and the Island of Malta in an additional four categories.

TABLE A41   MORTALITY FROM SPECIFIC DISEASES (NOT AGE-ADJUSTED)

Year	United States	Deaths per 100,000 Population	Sweden	England and Wales
Heart Disease				
1950	356		355	—
1955	357		337	311
1960	369		367	311
1965	367		411	—
1967	—		417	368
Cancer				
1950	140		164	—
1955	147		169	206
1960	149		182	215
1965	154		195	222
1967			199	228
Tuberculosis				
1950	23		39	35
1955	9		16	15
1960	6		8	8
1965	4		5	5
1967	4		4	4
Accidents[a]				
1950	61		38	37
1955	57		40	37
1960	52		42	39
1965	58		45	39
1967			43	39
Influenza and Pneumonia				
1950	31		53[b]	79

TABLE A41   MORTALITY FROM SPECIFIC DISEASES
(NOT AGE-ADJUSTED) (*Continued*)

Year	United States		Sweden	England and Wales
		Deaths per 100,000 Population		

Deaths per 100,000 Population

Year	United States		Sweden	England and Wales
1955	27		52[b]	54
1960	37		58[b]	56
1965	32		68[b]	69
1967	—		67[b]	68
		Suicide		
1950	11		15	10
1955	10		17	11
1960	11		19	11
1965	11		19	11
1967	11		23	10
		Homicide		
1950	5.3		—	0.7
1955	4.5		—	0.7
1960	4.7		—	0.6
1965	5.5		0.7	0.6
1967	6.3		0.8	0.6

Sources. United States: Bureau of the Census (1968), p. 58. Sweden: National Board of Health (1969), p. 154; National Central Bureau of Statistics (1968), pp. 288, 291. England and Wales: 1950, 1960 from Department of Health and Social Security (1969), p. 3; 1955 from Central Statistical Office (1965), p. 33; 1965, 1967 from Department of Health and Social Security (1969), p. 238. Includes operations of war.
[a]The 1966 automobile accident rate is 27 in the United States, 17 in Sweden, and 15 in England and Wales.
[b]Includes about 10 deaths per 100,000 population due to bronchitis.

Bibliography

Abel-Smith, Brian, "Labor's Social Plans," in *Socialism and Affluence; Four Fabian Essays*. London: Fabian Society, 1967.

———, *The Hospitals 1800–1948: A Study in Social Administration in England and Wales*. Cambridge: Harvard University Press, 1964.

———, *An International Study of Health Expenditure and Its Relevance for Health Planning*. Geneva: World Health Organization (Public Health Papers No. 32), 1967.

Abel-Smith, Brian and Richard M. Titmuss, *The Cost of the National Health Service in England and Wales*. Cambridge, England: Cambridge University Press (National Institute of Economic and Social Research, Occasional Papers, 18), 1956.

Agnell, Anna Lisa, "Øversikt av det Svenska Sjukhusväsendets Utveckling till 1900—talets Mitt," in *Svenska Sjukhusväsendets Utveckling till 1900—talets Mitt Tredje Delen*. Stockholm: Bokförlaget, Gothia, 1950. Pp. 27–87.

Åkerman, Nordal, *Apparaten Sverige*. Stockholm: Wahlström & Widstrand, 1970.

Albinsson, Gillis, *Public Health Services in Sweden*. Swedish Hospital Association, 1965.

Almond, Gabriel A. and Sidney Verba, *The Civic Culture; Political Attitudes and Democracy in Five Nations*. Princeton, N.J.: Princeton University Press, 1963.

American Hospital Association, *Hospitals, J.A.H.A.*, 43, 15 (August 1), 1969.

———, Hospitals, J.A.H.A., 44, 15, (August 1), 1970.

———, *Transactions of the 35th Annual Convention, Milwaukee*, September 11–15, 1933.

American Medical Association, *Distribution of Physicians, Hospitals, and Hospital Beds in the U.S.—1967*. Chicago: The Association, 1968.

249

Andersen, Ronald, *A Behavioral Model of Families' Use of Health Services*, Research Series No. 25. Chicago: Center for Health Administration Studies, University of Chicago, 1968.

Andersen, Ronald and Odin W. Anderson, *A Decade of Health Services: Social Survey Trends in Use and Expenditure*. Chicago: University of Chicago Press, 1967.

Andersen, Ronald, Björn Smedby, and Odin W. Anderson, *Medical Care Use in Sweden and the United States, A Comparative Analysis of Systems and Behavior*, Research Series No. 27. Chicago: Center for Health Administration Studies, University of Chicago, 1970.

Anderson, Odin W., "Hospital Charges in the United States," *Hospitals, J.A.H.A.*, May 16, 1957.

————, *The Uneasy Equilibrium; Private and Public Financing of Health Services in the United States, 1875–1965*. New Haven: College & University Press, 1968.

————, "Book Report," *Health Serv. Res.*, 3 (Spring 1968), 65–70.

Anderson, Odin W., Patricia Collette, and Jacob J. Feldman, *Changes in Family Medical Care Expenditures and Voluntary Health Insurance: A Five Year Resurvey*. Cámbridge: Harvard University Press, 1963.

Anderson, Odin W. and Jacob J. Feldman, *Family Medical Costs and Voluntary Health Insurance: A Nationwide Survey*. New York: McGraw-Hill, 1956.

Anderson, Odin W. and Joanna Kravits, *Health Services in the Chicago Area—A Framework for Use of Data*, Research Series No. 26. Chicago: Center for Health Administration Studies, University of Chicago, 1968.

Anderson, Odin W. and Monroe Lerner, *Measuring Health Levels in the United States, 1900–1958*, Research Series No. 11. New York: Health Information Foundation, 1960.

Anderson, Odin W. and Paul B. Sheatsley, *Comprehensive Medical Insurance—A Study of Costs, Use, and Attitudes Under Two Plans*, Research Series No. 9. Chicago: Center for Health Administration Studies, University of Chicago, 1959.

————, *Hospital Use—A Survey of Patient and Physician Decisions*, Research Series No. 24. Chicago: Center for Health Administration Studies, University of Chicago, 1967.

Andersson, Ingvar, *A History of Sweden*, translated from the Swedish by Carolyn Hannay. London: Weidenfeld and Nicolson, 1956.

Association of Chief Financial Officers in the Hospital Service in England and Wales, *Report of the Annual Conference*, Friday, October 15, 1954, 3, 3 (April, 1955).

Auster, Richard, Irving Leveson, and Deborah Sarachek, "The Production of Health; An Exploratory Study," *J. Human Resources*, 4 (Fall 1969), 411–436.

Bach, Pär-Erik, "How Sweden is Governed," in *Sweden in the Sixties*, Ingemar Wigelius, ed. Stockholm: Almquist and Wicksell, 1967. Pp. 49–71.

Backett, E. Maurice, "Community Medicine and the Improvement of Health Services; A Model for the University Contribution to Innovation," *Lancet*, 7610 (July 5, 1969).

Beveridge, Sir William, *Social Insurance and Allied Services*. New York: MacMillan Company, 1942.

Björkblom, Sixten, *Södermanslands Läns Landsting; Sammansättning Organisation, och Verksamhet*, Uppsala och Stockholm (Skrifter utgivna av Statsvetenskapliga Föreningen, Uppsala XIV), 1942.

Björkquist, Erik and Ivar Flygare, "Den Centrala Medicinal förvaltningen," in Wolfram Kock, ed., *Medicinalväsendet i Sverige, 1813–1962*. Stockholm: Nordiska Bokhandelns Förlag, 1963. Pp. 7–40.

Blau, Peter M., *Exchange and Power in Social Life*. New York: John Wiley and Sons, 1964.

Boorstin, Daniel J., *The Genius of American Politics*. Chicago: University of Chicago Press, 1953.

Borgenhammer, Edgar, *Makten över Sjukhuset*. Stockholm: Studieförbundet Näringsliv och Samhälle, 1968.

Bornet, Vaughn D., *Welfare in America*. Norman, Okla.: University of Oklahoma Press, 1960.

Braithwaite, William J., *Lloyd George's Ambulance Wagon; Being the Memoirs of William J. Braithwaite, 1911–1912*, edited with an introduction by Sir Henry N. Bunbury and with a commentary by Richard Titmuss. London: Methuen, 1957.

Brand, Jeanne L., *Doctors and the State: The British Medical Profession and Government Action in Public Health, 1870–1912*. Baltimore: Johns Hopkins Press, 1965.

British Medical Association, *Primary Medical Care*, Planning Unit Report No. 4. London: British Medical Association, 1970.

British Medical Journal, "Draft Interim Report of the Medical Planning Commission," 1, (1942), 743–753.

Bruno, Frank J., *Trends in Social Work as Reflected in the Proceedings of the National Conference of Social Work, 1874–1946*. New York: Oxford, 1948.

Brush, Frederick, M.D., Medical Superintendent, New York Post-Graduate Medical School and Hospital. Transactions of the American Hospital Association, 11th Annual Conference, XI, 1909.

Bunker, John P., "Surgical Manpower in the United States and in England and Wales," *New Engl. J. Med.*, 282, 3 (January 15, 1970), 135–143.

Bureau of the Census, *Statistical Abstract of the United States—1968, 1971*. Washington: U.S. Government Printing Office, 1968, 1971.

Carlsson, Sten, *Svensk Historia II: Tiden Efter 1718*. Stockholm: Svenska Bokförlaget, 1961.

———, *Bonde-Präst-Ämbetsman; Svensk Standscirkulation från 1680 till våre Dagar*. Stockholm: Bokförlaget Prisma, 1962.

Cartwright, Ann, *Patients and Their Doctors—A Study of General Practice.* London: Routledge & Kegan Paul, 1967.

Central Statistical Office, *Annual Abstract of Statistics, No. 102, 1965.* London: Her Majesty's Stationery Office, 1965.

————*Annual Abstract of Statistics,* No. 106, 1969, London: Her Majesty's Stationery Office, 1969.

————*Social Trends, A Publication of the Government Statistical Service,* Vol. 1, 1970, London: Her Majesty's Stationery Office, 1970.

Charney, Seth D., *Doctors: Surplus or Shortage,* unpublished, 1969.

Chester, T. E., *How Healthy Is the National Health Service?* District Board Review Reprint, 1968.

Clark, Colin, *The Conditions of Economic Progress,* Second Edition. London: MacMillan Company, 1951.

Cole, G. D. H. and Raymond Postgate, *The British Common People, 1746–1946.* London: Methuen (University Paperback), 1961.

Committee on Manpower Resources for Science and Technology, *The Brain Drain; Report of the Working Group on Migration.* London: Her Majesty's Stationery Office (command 3417), 1967.

Committee on the Civil Service, *Report,* Vol. 1. London: Her Majesty's Stationery Office (command 3638) (Lord Fulton, chairman), 1968.

Conant, Ralph W., *The Politics of Community Health,* Report of the Community Action Studies Project, National Commission on Community Health Services. Washington: Public Affairs Press, 1968.

Connery, Donald S., *The Scandinavians.* London: Eyre and Spottiswoode, 1966.

Corwin, E. A. C., *The American Hospital.* New York: Commonwealth Fund, 1946.

Crossman, R. H. S., article in *Socialism and Affluence; Four Fabian Essays.* London: Fabian Society, 1967.

Crozier, Michael, *The Bureaucratic Phenomenon.* Chicago: University of Chicago Press, 1964. P. 8.

Curwen, Michael and Brian Brookes, "Health Centers: Facts and Figures," *Lancet,* III, 7627 (1969).

Dagens Nyheter, February 9, 1970.

Dahl, Robert A., *Pluralistic Democracy in the United States—Conflict and Consent.* Chicago: Rand McNally, 1967.

Dahl, Robert A. and Charles E. Lindbloom, *Politics, Economics and Welfare.* New York: Harper, 1953.

Dahlström, Edmund, ed., *Svensk Samhälls Struktur i Sociologisk Belysning,* Third Edition. Stockholm: Svenska Bokförlaget/Norstedts, 1965.

de Grazia, Alfred and Ted Gurr, *American Welfare.* New York: New York University Press, 1961.

De Gré, Gerard, "Freedom and Social Structure," *Amer. Sociol. Rev.,* 11 (October 1946), 529–536.

De Tocqueville, Alexis, *Democracy in America,* edited and abridged by Richard D. Heffner. New York: New American Library, 1956.

Department of Health and Social Security, *Digest for Health Statistics for England and Wales, 1969.* London: Her Majesty's Stationery Office, 1969.

———*Digest of Health Statistics for England and Wales, 1970,* London: Her Majesty's Stationery Office, 1971.

———, *On the State of the Public Health, The Annual Report of the Chief Medical Officer of the Department of Health and Social Security for the Year 1968.* London: Her Majesty's Stationery Office, 1969.

———*Annual Report, 1970,* London: Her Majesty's Stationery Office, 1971.

———, *Adult Dental Health in England and Wales in 1968.* London: Her Majesty's Stationery Office, 1970.

———, *The Future of the National Health Services.* London: Her Majesty's Stationery Office, 1970.

de Schweinitz, Karl *England's Road to Social Security.* Philadelphia: University of Pennsylvania Press, 1943.

Dicey, A. V., *Lectures on the Relation Between Law and Public Opinion in England during the Nineteenth Century,* Second Edition. New York: MacMillan Company, 1963.

Diggory, Peter et al., "Preliminary Assessment of the 1967 Abortion Act in Practice," *Lancet,* 1, 7641 (February 7, 1970).

Division of Hospital and Medical Facilities, *Areawide Planning for Hospitals and Related Facilities—Report to the Joint Committee of the American Hospital Association and the Public Health Service,* U.S.P.H.S. Publication No. 855. Washington: U.S. Government Printing Office, 1961.

Dror, Yehezkel, "Comprehensive Planning: Common Fallacies Versus Preferred Features," in F. Van Schalgen, ed., *Essays in Honour of Professor Jac. P. Thijsse.* The Hague: Monton Co., 1967.

Dubos, Rene, *Mirage of Health, Utopias, Progress and Biological Change.* New York: Harper, 1959.

Eckstein, Harry, *Pressure Group Politics; The Case of the British Medical Association.* Stanford, Calif.: Stanford University Press, 1960.

———, *The English Health Service; Its Origins, Structure, and Achievements.* Cambridge: Harvard University Press, 1958.

———, "The British Political System," in Samuel H. Beer et al., *Patterns of Government; The Major Political Systems of Europe,* Second Edition, revised and enlarged. New York: Random House, 1962. Pp. 73–269.

Elvander, Nils, *Intresseorganisationerna i Dagens Sverige.* Lund: Gleerup, 1966.

Engel, Arthur, *Perspectives in Health Planning,* Health Clark Lectures, University of London. London: The Athlone Press, 1968.

Falk, I. J., Margaret Klem, and Nathan Sinai, *The Incidence of Illness and the Receipt and Cost of Medical Care among Representative Families; Experiences in Twelve Consecutive Months during 1928–1931,* Committee on the Costs of Medical Care No. 26. Chicago: University of Chicago Press, 1933.

Ferris, Paul, *The Doctors*. London: Gollancy, 1965.

First Secretary of State and Secretary of State for Economic Affairs, *The National Plan*. London: Her Majesty's Stationery Office (command 2764), 1965.

Flexner, Abraham, *Medical Education in the United States and Canada; A Report to the Carnegie Foundation for the Advancement of Teaching*, Bulletin No. 4. New York: Carnegie Foundation, 1910.

Forsyth, Gordon, *Doctors and State Medicine; A Study of the British Health Services*. Philadelphia: Lippincott, 1966.

Freyman, John G., "A Doctor Prescribes for the A.M.A.," *Harper's*, CCXXXI, August, 1965.

Friedman, Milton, *Capitalism and Freedom*. Chicago: University of Chicago Press, 1963.

Fry, John, *Medicine in Three Societies: A Comparison of Medical Care in the USSR, USA, and UK*. New York: American Elsevier Publishing Co., Inc., 1970.

Galbraith, John K., *The Affluent Society*. New York: Houghton-Mifflin, 1958.

Gilbert, Bentley B., *The Evolution of National Insurance in Great Britain: The Origins of the Welfare State*. London: Michael Joseph, Ltd., 1966.

Ginzberg, Eli, with Miriam Ostow, *Men, Money and Medicine*. New York: Columbia University Press, 1970.

Ginzberg, Eli, Dale L. Hiestand, and Beatrice G. Reubens, *The Pluralistic Economy*. New York: McGraw-Hill, 1965.

Glaser, William A., *Paying the Doctor; Systems of Remuneration and Their Effects*. Baltimore: Johns Hopkins Press, 1970.

Godber, George E., *The Future Place of the Personal Physician*, Michael M. Davis Lecture. Chicago: Center for Health Administration Studies, University of Chicago, 1969.

Gorer, Geoffrey, "What's the Matter with Britain?," *New York Times Magazine*, December 31, 1967.

Gregg, Pauline, *The Welfare State; An Economic and Social History of Great Britain from 1945 to the Present Day*. London: Harrap, 1967.

Grodzins, Morton, *The American System; A New View of Government in the United States*. Chicago: Rand McNally, 1966.

Harris, R. W., *National Health Insurance in Great Britain, 1911–1946*. London: Allen and Unwin, 1946.

Health Information Foundation, "A View of Our Family Physicians," *Progress in Health Services*, 1958.

Hedinger, Frederic R., *The Systems Approach to Health Services: A Framework*, Health Care Research Series No. 11. Iowa City: Graduate Program in Hospital Administration, 1969.

Hodgkinson, Ruth G., *The Origins of the National Health Service*. Los Angeles: University of California Press, 1967.

Höjer, Karl J., *Svensk Socialpolitisk Historia*. Stockholm: Norstedt, 1952.

Hunter, Floyd, *Top Leadership—U.S.A.* Chapel Hill: University of North Carolina, 1959.

Interdepartmental Committee to Coordinate Health and Welfare Activities, *The Nation's Health*. Washington: Government Printing Office, 1939.

Jewkes, John and Sylvia, *Value for Money in Medicine*. Oxford: Blackwell, 1963.

Johnson, T. L., editor and translator, *Economic Expansion and Structural Change; A Trade Union Manifesto*, Report Submitted to the 16th Congress of Landsorganisation i Sverige (The Swedish Federation of Trade Unions). London: Allen and Unwin, 1963.

Joint Commission on Mental Health and Illness, *Action for Mental Health*. New York: Science Editions, 1961.

Jones, Ivor, chairman, Advisory Panel, *Health Services Financing*. London: British Medical Association, 1970.

———, *Independent Medical Services, Ltd.*, mimeo, 1967.

Journal of the American Medical Association, **LXXIV** (May 1, 1920), 1319.

———, *Editorial*, **XCIII** (August 1929), 459.

———, *Editorial*, **XCIX** (December 3, 1932).

———, *Editorial*, **LXV** (November 20, 1951).

Journal of the American Pharmaceutical Association, 7 (October 1918), 900.

Katz, Daniel and Robert L. Kahn, *The Social Psychology of Organizations*. New York: John Wiley and Sons, 1966.

Kissick, William L., "Health Manpower in Transition," *Milbank Memorial Fund Quart.*, **XLVI**, 2 (January 1968).

Lane, Robert E., *Political Ideology; Why the American Common Man Believes What He Does*. Glencoe, Ill.: Free Press, 1962.

Lees, D. S., *Health Through Choice: An Economic Study of the British National Health Service*, Hobart Paper No. 14. London: Institute of Economic Affairs, 1961.

Lerner, Max, *America as a Civilization*. New York: Simon & Schuster, 1957.

Lerner, Monroe and Odin W. Anderson, *Health Progress in the United States, 1900–1960*. Chicago: University of Chicago Press, 1963.

Levy, Hermann, *National Health Insurance—A Critical Study*. Cambridge, England: Cambridge University Press, 1944.

Lindblom, Charles E., *The Intelligence of Democracy; Decision Making Through Mutual Adjustment*. New York: Free Press, 1965.

Lindeberg, Gösta, *Den Svenska Sjukkasserörelsens Historia*. Lund: 1949.

Lindencrona, Frederik, "Sjukvardblir hälsovård i förändligheteng samhälle," *Läkartidnengen*, 63 (September 21, 1966), 3549.

Lindsey, Almont, *Socialized Medicine in England and Wales; the National*

Health Service, 1948–1961. Chapel Hill, N.C.: University of North Carolina Press, 1962.

Lippman, Walter, *The Good Society; An Inquiry into the Principles of a Good Society.* New York: Little, Brown, and Co., 1937.

Lipset, Seymour M., *The First New Nation; The United States in Historical and Comparative Perspective.* New York: Basic Books, 1963.

Lowi, Theodore, *The End of Liberalism: Ideology, Policy, and the Crisis of Public Authority.* New York: Norton, 1969.

McConnell, Grant, *Private Power and American Democracy.* New York: Knopf, 1966.

McKenzie, Robert, *British Political Parties,* Second Edition. London: Mercury Books, 1963.

McKenzie, Robert and Allan Silver, *Angels in Marble; Working Class Conservatives in Urban England.* Chicago: University of Chicago Press, 1968.

McKeown, Thomas, *Medicine in Modern Society; Medical Planning Based on Evaluation of Medical Achievement.* New York: Hafner, 1966.

McNamara, Mary E. and Clifford Todd, "A Survey of Group Practice in the United States, 1969," *Amer. J. Public Health,* **60** (July 1970), 1305–1313.

McNeill, William H., *The Rise of the West, A History of the Human Community.* Chicago: University of Chicago Press, 1963.

McNerney, Walter J., *Hospital and Medical Economics: A Study of Population, Services, Costs, Methods of Payment, and Controls.* Chicago: Hospital Research and Educational Trust, 1962. (Two volumes.)

Mannheim, Karl, *Man and Society in an Age of Reconstruction.* New York: Harcourt, Brace, 1940.

Marquand, David, "The Dilemmas of 'Revisionist' Social Democracy," *Dissent,* November–December 1969.

Martin, J. P., *Social Aspects of Prescribing.* London: Heinemann, 1957.

May, Joel, *Health Planning; Its Past and Potential.* Chicago: Center for Health Administration Studies, University of Chicago, 1969.

Mechanic, David, "General Medical Practice in England and Wales; Its Organization and Future," *New Engl. J. Med.,* **279** (September 29, 1968), 668.

————, "General Practice in England and Wales: Results from a Survey of a National Sample of General Practitioners," *Med. Care,* **6** (May–June 1968), 253.

————, "Relevance of Experience in the English National Health Service to Medical Care in the United States: Some Comparisons and Contrasts," Department of Sociology, University of Wisconsin, unpublished paper, 1970.

Medical World News, "Legal Abortion Upsurge—Is the U. S. Ready?," December 26, 1969.

————"Two-Minute Abortion Is Here—Are We Ready?," May 12, 1972.

Mencher, Samuel, *British Private Medical Practice and the National Health Service.* Pittsburgh: University of Pittsburgh Press, 1968.

Miles, Arthur P., *An Introduction to Public Welfare*. Boston: Heath, 1949.

Mills, C. Wright, *The Power Elite*. New York: Oxford, 1956.

Ministry of Health, *A National Health Service*. London: Her Majesty's Stationery Office (command 6502), 1944.

————, *Annual Report of the Ministry of Health for the Year 1967*. London: Her Majesty's Stationery Office, 1968.

————, Consultative Council on Medical and Allied Services, Interim Report on the Future Provision of Medical and Allied Services. London: Her Majesty's Stationery Office (command 693), 1920.

————, *Report of the Committee of Enquiry into the Relationship of the Pharmaceutical Industry with the National Health Service, 1965–1967*. London: Her Majesty's Stationery Office (command 3410) (Lord Sainsbury, chairman), 1967.

————, Central Health Services Council Standing Medical Advisory Committee, *The Field Work of the Family Doctor, Report of the Family Doctor, Report of the Subcommittee*. London: Her Majesty's Stationery Office, 1963.

————, Committee on Cost of Prescribing, *Final Report*. London: Her Majesty's Stationery Office (Hinchliffe, chairman), 1959.

————(Department of Health for Scotland), Committee of Enquiry into the Cost of the National Health Service, *Report Presented to Parliament by the Minister of Health and the Secretary of State for Scotland*. London: Her Majesty's Stationery Office (command 9336), 1956.

————(Department of Health for Scotland), *Medical Staffing Structures in the Hospital Service*. London: Her Majesty's Stationery Office, 1961.

————(Department of Health for Scotland), *Report of the Committee on Senior Nursing Staff Structures*. London: Her Majesty's Stationery Office (Salmon, chairman), 1966.

————(Department of Health for Scotland), *Report of the Committee to Consider the Future Number of Medical Practitioners and the Appropriate Intake of Medical Students*. London: Her Majesty's Stationery Office (Willink, chairman), 1957.

Ministry of Housing and Local Government, *Management of Local Government—Report of the Committee* I. London: Her Majesty's Stationery Office, 1967.

Monsen, Joseph R. and Mark W. Cannon, *The Makers of Public Policy: American Power Groups and Their Ideologies*. New York: McGraw-Hill, 1965.

Moore, Barrington, *Social Origins of Dictatorship and Democracy; Lord and Peasant in the Making of the Modern World*. Boston: beacon Press, 1966.

Myrdal, Gunnar, "But Paradise Can Be Boring; The Swedish Way to Happiness," *New York Times Magazine*, January 30, 1966.

National Advisory Commission on Health Facilities, *Report to the President, December, 1968*. Washington: Government Printing Office, 1969.

National Advisory Commission on Health Manpower, *Report-Volume I*. Washington: Government Printing Office, November 1967.

National Board of Health, *Public Health in Sweden,* (1950, 1951, 1952, 1953, 1954, 1955, 1956, 1957, 1958, 1959, 1960, 1961, 1962, 1963, 1964, 1965, 1966, 1967). Stockholm: Official Statistics of Sweden: public health, 1952–1969.

National Center for Health Statistics, *Health Resources Statistics, 1968,* U.S. Department of Health, Education, and Welfare, 1968.

————, *Monthly Vital Statistics Report,* Vol. 17, No. 12, "Advance Report— Final Mortality Statistics, 1967," March 25, 1969.

————, *Monthly Vital Statistics Report,* Vol. 18, No. 9, "Estimated Annual Volume of Dental Visits in the United States, 1968," December 1969.

————, *Monthly Vital Statistics Report,* Vol. 18, No. 11, "Advance Report—Final Natality Statistics, 1968," January 30, 1970.

————, Series 3, No. 6, *International Comparison of Perinatal and Infant Mortality, the United States and Six West European Countries,* U.S. Department of Health, Education, and Welfare, 1967.

————, Series 10, No. 39, *Prescribed and Non-prescribed Medicines, United States, July, 1964–June, 1965,* U.S. Department of Health, Education, and Welfare, 1967.

————, Series 10, No. 49, *Volume of Physician Visits, United States, July, 1966–June, 1967,* U.S. Department of Health, Education, and Welfare, 1968.

————, Series 21, No. 11, *Natality Statistics Analysis—United States, 1964,* U.S. Department of Health, Education, and Welfare, 1967.

————, *Vital Statistics of the United States—1967,* Volume II, Mortality, Part A, U.S. Department of Health, Education, and Welfare, 1969.

————, *Vital Statistics of the United States—1967,* Volume II, Mortality, Part B, U.S. Department of Health, Education, and Welfare, 1969.

National Central Bureau of Statistics, *Statistical Abstract of Sweden.* The Bureau: Stockholm, 1968.

National Commission on Community Health Services, *Health Is a Community Affair.* Cambridge: Harvard University Press, 1966.

National Health Service, *A Hospital Plan for England and Wales.* London: Her Majesty's Stationery Office (command 1604), 1962.

————, *The Hospital Building Programme; A Revision of the Hospital Plan for England and Wales.* London: Her Majesty's Stationery Office (command 3000), 1966.

National Institute of Mental Health, *Patients in Mental Institutions (1965), Part III, Private Mental Hospitals and General Hospitals with Psychiatric Service.* Washington: U.S. Department of Health, Education, and Welfare, 1968.

Navarro, Vicente, "Planning Personal Health Services: A Markovian Model," *Med. Care,* 7 (May–June 1969), 242–249.

Nicholson, Max, *The System; The Misgovernment of Modern Britain.* London: Hodder and Stoughton, 1967.

Nilsson, Göran B., *100 Års Landstingspolitik; Västmanlands Länslandsting, 1863–1963*. Published by Västmanlands Länslandsting, 1966.

Office of Health Economics, "The Cost of National Health Services," *OHE Information Sheet*, No. 5, January 1969.

Orwell, George, *The English People*. London: Collins, 1947.

Paige, Deborah and Kit Jones, *Health and Welfare Services in Britain in 1975*. Cambridge, England: Cambridge University Press, 1966.

Pelling, Henry, *The Origins of the Labour Party, 1880–1900*. London: MacMillan Company, 1954.

————, *A History of British Trade Unionism*. Middlesex: Penguin Books, 1963.

Peterson et al., "What is Value for Money in Medical Care," *Lancet*, 1, 7493 (April 8, 1967), 771–775.

Pinker, Robert, *English Hospital Statistics, 1861–1938*. London: Heinemann, 1966.

polanyi, Karl, *The Great Transformation*. New York: Farrar and Rinehart, 1944.

Powell, J. Enoch, *A New Look at Medicine and Politics*. London: Pitman, 1966.

President's Commission on Heart Disease, Cancer and Stroke, *A National Program to Conquer Heart Disease, Cancer and Stroke*. Washington: U.S. Government Printing Office, 1964.

President's Commission on the Health Needs of the Nation, *Building America's Health*. Washington: U.S. Government Printing Office, 1952, 5 volumes.

Reed, Louis S. and Ruth S. Hanft, "National Health Expenditures, 1950–1964," *Soc. Secur. Bull.*, 29, 1 (January 1966).

Reed, Louis S. and Dorothy P. Rice, "Private Medical Care Expenditures and Voluntary Health Insurance, 1948–1961," *Soc. Secur. Bull.*, 25, 11 (November 1962).

Rein, Martin, "Social Class and the Health Service," *New Society*, 379 (November 20, 1969).

Rice, Dorothy and Barbara Cooper, "National Health Expenditures, 1960–1966," *Soc. Secur. Bull.*, 31, 4 (April 1968).

————, "National Health Expenditures in 1929–1968," *Soc. Secur. Bull.*, 33, 1 (January 1970).

Riesman, David, *The Lonely Crowd*. New Haven: Yale University Press, 1950.

Rose, Arnold, *The Power Structure; Political Process in American Society*. New York: Oxford, 1967.

Rose, Richard, *Politics in England*. New York: Little, Brown & Co., 1964.

Rosén, Jerker, *Svensk Historia I: Tiden Före 1718*. Stockholm: Svenska Bokförlaget, 1962.

Rosenfeld, Alvin, "Private Group Practice in Sweden," *Med. Care*, 7 (January–February 1969), 62–71.

Rosenthal, Albert H., *The Social Programs of Sweden; A Search for Security in a Free Society*. Minneapolis: University of Minnesota Press, 1967.

Royal Commission on Doctors' and Dentists' Remuneration, 1957–1960, *Report to Parliament, February, 1960*. London: Her Majesty's Stationery Office (command 939), 1960.

Royal Commission on Medical Education, 1965–1968, *Report*. London: Her Majesty's Stationery Office (command 3569), 1968.

Royal Commission on National Health Insurance. London: Her Majesty's Stationery Office (command 2596), 1926.

Royal Commission on the Poor Laws and the Relief of Distress. London: Her Majesty's Stationery Office (command 4499), 1909.

Runciman, W. G., *Relative Deprivation and Social Justice: A Study of Attitudes to Social Inequality in Twentieth Century England*. Berkeley, Calif.: University of California Press, 1966.

Sampson, Anthony, *Anatomy of Britain Today*. New York: Harper and Row, 1965.

Schmidt, Folke and Stig Strömholm, *Legal Values in Modern Sweden*. Stockholm: Svenska Bokförlaget Norstedts-Bonniers, 1964.

Schultze, Charles L., *Political Bargaining, Systematic Analysis and Federal Budget Decisions*. Washington: Brookings Institutions Research Report No. 95, 1969.

Schumpeter, Joseph A., *Capitalism, Socialism, and Democracy*, Third Edition. New York: Harper Torch Books, 1962.

Secretary, Department of Health, Education, and Welfare, *Report of the Task Force on Medicaid and Related Programs*. Washington: Government Printing Office, 1970.

Secretary's Advisory Committee on Hospital Effectiveness, *Report*, U.S. Department of Health, Education, and Welfare, 1968.

Seldon, Arthur, *After the NHS; Reflections on the Development of Private Health Insurance in Britain in the 1970's*. London: Institute of Economic Affairs, Occasional Paper 21, 1968.

———, *Taxation and Welfare*. London: Institute of Economic Affairs, Research Monograph No. 14, 1967.

Seldon, Arthur and Hamish Gray, *Universal or Selective Social Benefits*. London: Institute of Economic Affairs, Research Monograph No. 8, 1967.

Shils, Edward A., "On Science and the Polity," *Social Science Research Council*, XV, 1, Pt. 2 (March 1961).

Shonfield, Andrew, "In the Course of Investigation," *New Society*, No. 356 (July 24, 1969), 123–125.

———, *Modern Capitalism: The Changing Balance of Public and Private Power*. London: Oxford University Press, 1969.

Shryock, Richard H., *The Development of Modern Medicine*. London: Gollancz, 1948.

Skidelsky, Robert, *Politicians and the Slump*. New York: MacMillan Company, 1967.

Skidmore, Max J., *Medicare and the American Rhetoric of Reconciliation*. University, Ala.: University of Alabama Press, 1970.

Social Security Administration, *The Size and Shape of the Medical Care Dollar*. Washington: U.S. Department of Health, Education, and Welfare, 1969.

Somers, Herman M. and Anne R., *Medicare and the Hospitals; Issues and Prospects*. Washington: Brookings Institution, 1967.

Southwick, Arthur F., *The Doctor, The Hospital and the Patient in England, Rights and Responsibilities under National Health Service*. Ann Arbor: Bureau of Business Research, Graduate School of Business Administration, University of Michigan, 1968.

Statens Öffentliga Utredninga, *Bättre Aldringsvård, Sjukhem—Bostader—Hemhjälp*, 5, 1964.

———, *Den Öppna Läkarvarden: Riket Utredning och Förslag av Medicinalstyrelsen*, 14, 1948.

———, *Förvaltning och Folkstyre; Betänkande av Länsdemokratiutredningen*, 47, 1968.

———, *Hälso-och Socialvårdens Centrala Administration, Betänkande avgivet av Socialstyrelseutredningen och MCA-Utredningen*.

———, *Läkemedelsförmånen av 1961 Års Sjukförsäkringsutrednings Betänkande II*, 28, 1966.

———, *Läkemedelsförsörjning i Samverkan Betankande Angivet av Läkemedelsförsörjningsutredningen*, 46, 1969.

———, *Mentalsjukhusens Personal Organisation, Del II, Målsättning och Utformning*, 50, 1965.

———, *Nytt Skattesystem*, 25, 1964.

———, *Om Läkarbehov och Läkartillgång, Betånkande av Läkarprognos Utredningen*, 8, 1961.

———, *Riksplan för Samarbete Inom Specialiserad Sjukhusvård av Särskilt Tillkallad Utredningsmä*, 26, 1958.

———, *Sjukhus och Öppen Vård*, 1963.

———, *Sjuksköterske Utbildningen I. Grundutbildning. Betänkande av 1962 Års Utedning Angående Sjuksköterske Utbildningen*, 45, 1964.

———, *Tandvårdsforsäkring*, 1961 Års Sjukforsäkringsutredning Betänkande I, 4, 1965.

———, *Utredningar och Förslag Angående Lag om Allmän Sjukförsäkring*, 15, 1944.

Stein, Herbert, *The Fiscal Revolution in America*. Chicago: University of Chicago Press, 1969.

Stern, Berhard J., *American Medical Practice in the Context of a Century*. New York: Commonwealth Fund, 1945.

Stevens, Rosemary, *Medical Practice in Modern England, The Impact of Specialization and State Medicine*. New Haven: Yale University Press, 1966.

Stewart, William and Philip E. Enterline, "Effects of the N.H.S. on Physician Utilization and Health in England and Wales," *New Engl. J. Med.*, 265 (December 14, 1961), 1194.

Sundquist, James L., *Politics and Policy; The Eisenhower, Kennedy and Johnson Years.* Washington: Brookings Institution, 1968.

Surgeon General's Consultant Group on Nursing, *Toward Quality Nursing— Needs and Goals*, U.S.P.H.S. Publication No. 992. Washington: U.S. Government Printing Office, 1963.

Sutton, Francis X. et al., *American Business Creed.* Cambridge: Harvard University Press, 1956.

Svenska Läkartidningen, "Arbetstidsfrågan det största problemet i sluttasen," 66 (1970), 923–930.

————, "Betänkande angående en reformerad sjukförsäkring," 27 (nr. 3) 87 (1930).

————, "Centralstyrelsensyttrande i sjukkassefrågan," 27, 1598 (1930).

————, "Debatt viktig om enhetstaxan," 66, (1969), 662.

————, "Det nya förslaget om ersättning för läkarvard," 66 (1969), 1202–1207.

————, "Läkarna begär ingen fördubblad lön; parterna ense om oförandrad inkomst," 66 (1969), 4625–4628.

————, "Läkarnas uppgifter till sjukkassorna över meddelad läkarvård," 36 (nr. 9), 462 (1939).

————, "Lagen om allmän sjukförsakring, Sveriges Läkarforbunds yttrande över social vårdskommittens betänkande," 41 (nr. 40), 2361 (1944).

————, "Risk att målet förfelas ökat tryck på sjukvården," 66, (1969), 2123–2132.

————, "Ytterligare några remissytranden angående socialvårdskommittens betankande," 42 (nr. 5), 241 (1945).

————, "Läkarforbundets remissyttrande över Höjerska förslaget," 46 (nr. 3) 109 (1949).

The Observer, Editorial, London, April 26, 1970.

Tingsten, Herbert, *Den Svenska Social Democratiens Idéutvekling.* Sttockholm: Tidens Förlag, 1941.

Titmuss, Richard M., *Commitment to Welfare.* New York: Panthenon Books, 1968.

————, *Problems of Social Policy.* London: Her Majesty's Stationery Office, 1950.

Tomasson, Richard F., *Sweden: Prototype of the Modern Society.* New York: Random House, 1970.

————, "The Extraordinary Success of the Swedish Social Democrats," *J. Polit.*, 31, (1969), 772–798.

Townsend, Peter, "Does Selectivity Mean a Nation Divided," introduction to

Social Security for All? Eleven Fabian Essays. London: Fabian Society, 1968.

Tuchman, Barbara, *The Proud Tower; A Portrait of the World Before the War, 1890–1914.* New York: MacMillan Company, 1966.

Uhr, Carl G., *Sweden's Social Security System; An Appraisal of Its Economic Impact in the Postwar Period,* Research Report No. 14. Washington: U.S. Government Printing Office, Office of Research and Statistics, Social Security Amdinistration, 1966.

United Nations, *Demographic Yearbook—1949–1950.* New York: United Nations Publishing Service, 1951.

————, *Demographic Yearbook—1967.* New York: United Nations Publishing Service, 1968.

United States Congress, House of Representatives, Committee on Ways and Means, 87th Congress, First Session, Vols 1–4, *Health Services for the Aged under the Social Security Insurance System: Hearings Before the Committee.* Washington: u.S. Government Printing Office, 1961.

————, Senate, Committee on the Judiciary, Subcommittee on Antitrust and Monopoly, 87th Congress, First Session, *Administered Prices, Drugs— Report of the Committee.* Washington: U.S. Government Printing Office, 1961.

Vaughan, Paul, *Doctors' Commons; A Short History of the British Medical Association.* London: Heineman, 1954.

Viorst, Milton, "There Is No Raymond Aron Cult; Talk with a Reasonable Man," *New York Times Magazine,* April 19, 1970.

Wagner, Carruth J., "Program Planning: A Process of Health Program Planning and Implementation," *Arch. Environ. Health,* 12 (May 1969), 660–669.

Wawrinsky, Richard, *Sveriges Lasaretts-väsende förr och nu, ett Styck Svensk kulturhistoria.* Stockholm: Författarens Förlag, 1906.

Webb, Beatrice, *Our Partnership,* edited by Barbara Drake and Margaret I. Cole. New York: Longmans, Green, 1948.

Weber, Max, *The Protestant Ethic and the Spirit of Capitalism,* translated by Talcott Parsons with a foreword by Richard H. Tawney. New York: Scribner, 1958.

————, *The Theory of Social and Economic Organization,* translation by A. M. Henderson and Talcott Parsons, edited with an introduction by Talcott Parsons. Glencoe, Ill.: Free Press, 1964.

Wildavsky, Aaron, *The Politics of the Budgetary Process.* Boston: Little, Brown & Co., 1964.

Wilensky, Harold L. and Charles N. Lebeaux, *Industrial Society and Social Welfare.* New York: Russell Sage Foundation, 1958.

Willcocks, A. J., *The Creation of the National Health Service; A Study of Pressure Groups and a Major Social Policy Decision.* London: Routledge and Kegan Paul, 1967.

Williams, Robin, *American Society; A Sociological Interpretation*. New York: Knopf, 1960.

Young, Michael, *The Rise of Meritocracy, 1870–2033; An Essay on Education and Equality*. Harmondsworth, England: Penguin Books, 1958.

Zetterberg, Hans L., "Traditioner och möjligheter i Nordisk Sociologi," *Sociologisk Forskning*, **III**, 1 (1966), 1–21.

Zweig, Ferdynand, *The Worker in an Affluent Society*. London: Heinemann, 1961.

Index of Authors

265

Silver, Allan, 94n, 163n
Sinai, Nathan, 67n
Skidelsky, Robert, 163n
Skidmore, Max J., 97n
Smedby, Björn, 113n, 133n, 135n, 143n,
    149n, 159n, 187n, 240n
Somers, Anne R., 97n
Somers, Herman M., 97n
Southwick, Arthur F., 108n
Stern, Berhard J., 51n
Stevens, Rosemary, 124n
Stewart, William, 192n
Stromholm, Stig, 163n
Sundquist, James L., 97n
Sutton, Francis, 163n

Tingsten, Herbert, 42n
Titmuss, Richard M., 60, 64, 84, 90n, 163n,
    169–170, 201, 213n, 218n–219n
Todd, Clifford, 198n
Tomasson, Richard F., 163n
Townsend, Peter, 201, 204

Trevelyan, G. M., 55n
Truman, Harry, 71–72
Tuchman, Barbara, 55, 163n

Uhr, Carl G., 163n

Verba, Sidney, 162–163
Viorst, Milton, 30n

Wagner, Carruth J., 9n
Wawrinsky, Richard, 40n, 43n
Webb, Beatrice, 55–56, 58, 63, 67, 85
Webb, Sidney, 55–56, 67, 85
Weber, Max, 27, 31n
Wildavsky, Aaron, 29n
Wilensky, Harold L., 31n
Willcocks, A. J., 82n, 87
Williams, Robin, 163n

Young, Michael, 94n, 163n

Zetterberg, Hans L., 163n
Zweig, Ferdinand, 163n

Index of Subjects

Index of Other Sources

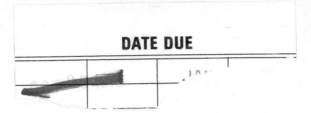